INTRAOPERATIVE AND
LAPAROSCOPIC ULTRASONOGRAPHY

Intraoperative and Laparoscopic Ultrasonography

O. JAMES GARDEN
BSc, MD, FRCSGlas, FRCSEd
Senior Lecturer in Surgery and Honorary Consultant
University Department of Surgery
Royal Infirmary, Edinburgh

With contributions by
J. DONALD GREIG
MB, ChB, FRCSEd

TIMOTHY G. JOHN
MB, ChB, FRCSEd

W. ANTHONY MILES
MB, ChB, FRCSEd

SIMON PATERSON-BROWN
MPh, MS, FRCSEng, FRCSEd

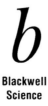

**Blackwell
Science**

© 1995 by
Blackwell Science Ltd
Editorial Offices:
Osney Mead, Oxford OX2 0EL
25 John Street, London WC1N 2BL
23 Ainslie Place, Edinburgh EH3 6AJ
238 Main Street, Cambridge
  Massachusetts 02142, USA
54 University Street, Carlton
  Victoria 3053, Australia

Other Editorial Offices:
Arnette Blackwell SA
1, rue de Lille, 75007 Paris
France

Blackwell Wissenschafts-Verlag GmbH
  Kurfürstendamm 57
  10707 Berlin, Germany

  Feldgasse 13, A-1238 Wien
  Austria

First published 1995

Set by Setrite Typesetters Ltd, Hong Kong
Printed and bound in the UK by
Cambus Litho Ltd, East Kilbride

DISTRIBUTORS

Marston Book Services Ltd
PO Box 87
Oxford OX2 0DT
(*Orders:* Tel: 01865 791155
       Fax: 01865 791927
       Telex: 837515)

North America
  Blackwell Science, Inc.
  238 Main Street
  Cambridge, MA 02142
  (*Orders:* Tel: 800 215-1000
            617 876-7000
        Fax: 617 492-5263)

Australia
  Blackwell Science Pty Ltd
  54 University Street
  Carlton, Victoria 3053
  (*Orders:* Tel: 03 347-0300
         Fax: 03 349-3016)

Records for this title
are available from the British Library
and the Library of Congress

ISBN 0-632-03553-6

Contents

Contributors

O. JAMES GARDEN BSc, MD, FRCSGlas, FRCSEd
Senior Lecturer in Surgery and Honorary Consultant, University Department of
Surgery, Royal Infirmary, Edinburgh

J. DONALD GREIG MB, ChB, FRCSEd
Senior Registrar, University Department of Surgery, Royal Infirmary, Edinburgh

TIMOTHY G. JOHN MB, ChB, FRCSEd
Lecturer, University Department of Surgery, Royal Infirmary, Edinburgh

W. ANTHONY MILES MB, ChB, FRCSEd
Surgical Registrar, Western General Hospital, Edinburgh

SIMON PATERSON-BROWN MPh, MS, FRCSEng, FRCSEd
Consultant Surgeon, Royal Infirmary, Edinburgh

Preface

It is the aim of this book to provide the general surgeon and the radiologist with an insight into the potential applications of ultrasonography in the operating theatre. Clearly, any such text will struggle to cover all the possible uses of ultrasound during surgery and, for this reason, no attempt has been made to encompass the more specialist applications such as in the fields of vascular surgery and neurosurgery.

There has been a reluctance amongst surgeons to consider the routine use of ultrasonography in their surgical practice. Perhaps the concern that the lifting of an ultrasound probe would lead to a demarcation dispute with radiological colleagues has contributed to their reluctance to grapple with this technological advance. It is clear, however, from the experience of gynaecologists, vascular surgeons and urologists that diagnostic ultrasound can be applied safely in their own clinical practices and benefit the patient considerably.

Intraoperative ultrasonography has had a number of enthusiastic champions in the past, but has only proved popular in the Far East and on the European Continent. Surgeons in these countries have been convinced of the value of this investigative modality in their own specialist and general surgical fields. The interest shown in the technique had increased by the end of the 1980s but it has taken the arrival of laparoscopic surgery to demonstrate to the minimally invasive surgeon that intraoperative and laparoscopic ultrasonography have much to offer in the investigation and treatment of intra-abdominal disease.

O. J. Garden

Acknowledgements

This book would not have been possible without the help of a number of individuals.

I will forever be indebted to Professor Henri Bismuth and Professor Denis Castaing for having first introduced me to intraoperative ultrasonography during my attachment in their unit in Paris. I must acknowledge the guidance afforded to me over the years by Professor David Carter, Regius Professor in Surgery, Royal Infirmary, Edinburgh. He has been an excellent mentor to me and I am indebted to him for allowing me to develop my own specialist skills under his charge.

I would like also to acknowledge the help afforded to me over the years by colleagues and, in particular, the theatre nursing staff, who, under the direction of Jenny Kennedy, have shown extreme patience with us. Without their presence and support we would have been unable to develop so many 'expert' ultrasonographers. Special thanks are due to Tim John who has managed to survive the explosion of interest in laparoscopic ultrasonography. His help in assembling the illustrations and scans has been much appreciated.

I thank my wife, Amanda, and my two children, Stephen and Katie, for puting up with my long absences from home. Their support and understanding has been immense.

I would like to dedicate this book to the memory of my father, James Garden, who was right to guide me away from his chosen career in orthopaedics. I am sorry that he is not here to share in my modest successes.

I sincerely hope that this book will show the potential of ultrasound in modern surgical practice. It is a technique, the skill for which has been readily acquired by my junior surgical colleagues, some of whom have kindly given their time and experience towards the preparation of this book. I hope that the reader will be able to appreciate the enormous potential of this technology and be able to develop a place for it in their own practice.

O. J. Garden

1: Basics and General Principles of Intraoperative and Laparoscopic Ultrasound

Introduction

Developments over recent years have been such that compact and robust ultrasound machines are now readily available for use in the operating theatre. These instruments can provide high-resolution images and can display instant movement of the ultrasound transducer or of the structures being examined.

Although a detailed explanation of the fundamentals of ultrasound and its applications is beyond the scope of this chapter, the basic principles are outlined to enable the surgeon to make effective use of and interpret the images obtained in the operating theatre.

Theory

Ultrasonography is dependent on the physical properties of piezoelectric crystals. The shape of the crystal changes when an electric is applied, and, conversely, a mechanical altering of its shape generates a weak electric current. These crystals can therefore be used to transmit and receive ultrasound signals. Application of a high-frequency electric current can cause the crystal to vibrate and create sound waves outwith the range of the human ear. If the crystal is subjected to high-frequency sound waves, a small alternating electric current is produced at the same frequency as the amplitude of the sound wave and in direct proportion to it. Varying the frequency of the electric current acting on the crystal may control the frequency of the sound, and to achieve the most efficient signal production the crystals must vibrate at a frequency that produces the greatest intensity.

Types of ultrasound

Ultrasound consists of mechanical waves with alternating regions of high and low pressure propagating through a medium. In diagnostic ultrasonography, the ultrasound waves oscillate at frequencies from 3.5 to 10 MHz or millions of cycles per second. The velocity of ultrasound waves is dependent on the medium through which they propagate, with this being lowest in air and highest in bone. The velocity of these waves in the soft tissues is almost identical to that of water.

The two main types of diagnostic ultrasound in principal use at the present time are *imaging reflective ultrasound* and *Doppler ultrasound velocity detection.*

Doppler ultrasound

The Doppler effect is a change in the apparent frequency of a sound when either the receiver or the source is in motion relative to the other. The application of this effect can therefore detect motion within the tissues. The detected frequency will increase as the distance between the source and receiver decreases. Similarly, the frequency is decreased as the distance increases. A frequency shift will be produced if a reflector is positioned between the source and the receiver and if it increases or decreases the sound-path distance between the two structures. If both the ultrasound source and the receiver are stationary, the velocity of the reflector will determine the degree of the frequency shift. This principle is used to measure blood flow with the blood itself acting as the reflector.

When two piezoelectric transducers are mounted in proximity to one another, one can serve as the source of ultrasound (transmitter), whilst the other can act as the receiver. The transducers can detect motion in the tissues if they are angled slightly. The pulsation of the vessel walls or the return in the direction of the sound source (back scattering) from the blood cells produces reflection. The resultant difference in the frequency between transmitted and received signals is detected either as an audible signal or an analogue display on a monitor. This frequency shift will increase the greater the velocity of the blood with respect to the transducers.

Imaging reflective ultrasound

Diagnostic imaging ultrasound is based on two types of reflection that are determined by the wavelength of the ultrasound beam and the size of the reflector. Specular reflection occurs when sound waves passing through one medium strike a surface or object of a different medium that has a dimension larger than the wavelength of the sound beam itself. An example of specular reflection is the reflection of a beam of light from a mirror (Fig. 1.1). The detector would have to be positioned in the line of reflection to sense the beam.

Scattering will arise if the object or surface of a different medium is of a smaller dimension than the wavelength of the incident sound beam (Fig. 1.2). Sound waves are sent in a number of directions and some may return in the direction of the sound source. Small objects that pass in the sound beam, such as blood coursing through a vessel, typically produce this back scattering. Scattering may also arise when the sound beam strikes an irregular surface. Whereas specular reflection would occur if the surface is smooth, the rough surface scatters the sound energy in a number of different directions. This weakens the sound intensity in any particular direction and distinguishes scattering from specular reflection where the reflected sound intensity is maintained.

In imaging reflective ultrasound a piezoelectric transducer acts both as a transmitter and as a receiver (Fig. 1.3). The transducer acts as a transmitter

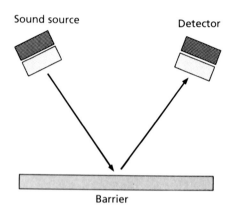

Fig. 1.1 Specular reflection demonstrated as a sound beam arising from a sound source, reflected by a barrier as an identical beam that is sensed by the detector.

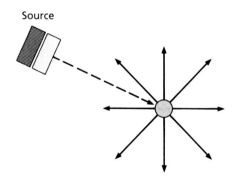

Fig. 1.2 Scattering demonstrated by the reflection of sound waves. These have passed in a number of directions after striking a small object.

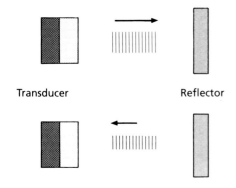

Transducer   Reflector

Fig. 1.3 Principles of imaging reflective ultrasound. The transducer transmits a short pulse of ultrasound, which when it strikes the reflector returns as a weaker signal to the transducer that is now acting as a receiver.

Fig. 1.4 Laparoscopic ultrasound scan demonstrating a linear hyperechoic line between the right kidney (RK) and the liver on which the ultrasound probe has been placed. This line represents the peritoneum and Gerota's fascia, which envelopes the kidney. GB, gallbladder.

for a short period and converts to receiver mode for a longer period. This is necessary to allow sufficient time for the transmitted sound pulse to be reflected back to the transducer. The cycle of pulse transmissions and receptions varies from 1000 to 8000 pulses per second, but the higher this repetition rate the poorer the penetration into the tissues. This effect is of great significance when one considers the advantages of operative ultrasound probes, which do not require the same penetration as transabdominal probes and as a result produce images of high resolution.

The transmission and reception of a sound pulse provide information that is dependent on the energy intensity or amplitude of the reflected signal or echo, the time taken for transmission and reflection, and the rate of change of this time duration if the cause of this echo is in motion. The amount of sound reflected at the interface between two media will be determined by the difference between their acoustic impedance, which is determined by the density and the velocity at which the sound is propagated through the medium. If the two media had similar acoustic impedance as might arise, for example, when a tumour of similar echogenicity is being examined in the liver, there is no reflection of the ultrasound beam between the two structures and the boundary, or limits of the tumour may not be apparent. On the other hand, if there is a substantial difference between the acoustic impedance of the two media, more sound is reflected back. A good example of this on an ultrasound scan would be the reflection from the interface of fascia between the liver and the kidney (Fig. 1.4).

It should be appreciated that the tissue under examination can absorb sound energy which may be lost as heat. This effect is related to the viscosity of the structure under examination and to the frequency of the sound waves. The higher the frequency, the greater the absorption is likely to be. In practical terms, lower frequency ultrasound transducers are employed to improve the penetration of the tissues. The surgeon can employ routinely operative ultrasound probes of higher frequency because tissue penetration

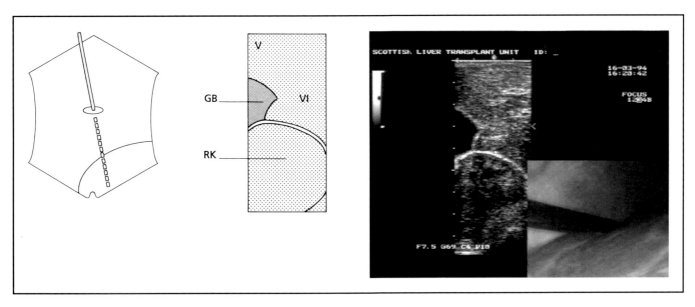

(through the abdominal wall) is of lesser importance than producing an image of high quality or resolution.

Loss of the intensity of the sound signal as it passes through tissue is called attenuation. It is dependent not only on the distance the beam of sound requires to pass through the tissues, but also on the extent of specular reflection, scattering, absorption and spreading of the ultrasound beam. Most ultrasound machines will employ a technique of amplifying more distant signals during the time taken between pulse transmission and the return of the echo. Echoes that have to travel a greater distance between propagation and return, therefore, undergo greater attenuation than echoes that take less time. In ultrasound machines that employ this form of time-gain compensation, the amplitude boost given to the returning echoes provides a more realistic indicator of the echogenicity of the structure responsible for reflecting the echoes.

Ultrasound systems

There have been considerable developments in ultrasound equipment over recent years and only a brief description is given of the earlier systems, some features of which are maintained in newer equipment. These can be broadly divided into one-dimensional and two-dimensional systems.

One-dimensional systems

In A-mode ultrasonography the monitor shows the position of the interface producing the echo as a spike (Fig. 1.5). The greater the reflected energy, the greater the height reached by the spike. Several spikes may be observed if more than one reflector is present. A-mode imaging can measure the distance and attenuation along the path of ultrasound transmission and reflection.

In M-mode ultrasonography time-sequence recording determines the rate of change of a moving reflector in one dimension, which is similar to A-mode except that the image is processed over time. Clinicians can employ M-mode scanning to study the motion of objects such as a heart valve.

Two-dimensional systems

Two-dimensional reflective ultrasound is known as B-mode imaging. An aggregation of lines of ultrasound transmission and reflection produces the two-dimensional image. These lines comprise dots of varying brightness that depict the amplitude intensity from the reflection of ultrasound waves. If an image is to be seen in two dimensions, a single transducer or multiple transducers must be moved to visualise the subject and this is termed scanning.

The images obtained on scanning can be restricted to display the extremes of reflectivity on the one hand, and absence of reflection on the other.

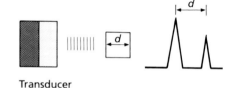

Transducer

Fig. 1.5 A transmitted sound wave produces two amplitude spikes as it passes towards an object. The distance (d) between the spikes is identical to the size of the object (A-mode).

The monitor would display these as bright echoes or dark areas of sonolucency. In practical terms such assessment of the tissues would provide the clinician with limited information and so the different degrees of echoity or echogenicity are seen as various shades of grey. This gives rise to the term of grey-scale B-mode imaging, which has now moved from compound to real-time B-mode scanning.

In compound B-mode scanning a single transducer produces a two-dimensional image on a cathode ray tube that has the capacity to store the image. The transducer produces a line across the monitor and the successive development of lines constructs an image. In this system an arm links the transducer to allow sensors to track the position of the transducer. This type of imaging system is cumbersome and real-time scanning has superseded it.

Abdominal and operative ultrasonography use real-time imaging. A linear array of transducers or an automatic (mechanical) sector scan provides an electronic image in near instant time (Fig. 1.6). In sector scanning a pie-shaped image is obtained as an ultrasound beam sweeps a sector. This is achieved either by the use of a motor-driven transducer or by means of phased array transducers. A monitor screen displays each real-time frame which changes over 30 times per second. The rapid sequence of images presents real-time motion.

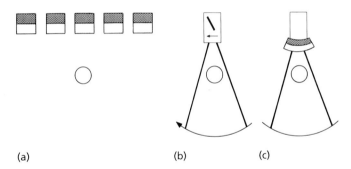

Fig. 1.6 A battery of crystals transmit and receive their own pulses to produce a linear-array scan (a). A motor oscillates in the transducer through a sector (b). A phased array of transducers electronically causes an ultrasound beam to sweep a sector to produce an image (c).

(a)   (b)   (c)

Real-time imaging may detect motion in the tissues or this may be produced by displacement of the transducer itself. Pulsation of blood vessels or movement of blood within them may be visible and is useful in differentiating them from other tubular structures such as the bile duct in the porta hepatis. Movement of the transducer enables the clinician to explore a structure in detail, almost building a three-dimensional view of the organ. Real-time imaging is a dynamic investigation which is difficult to demonstrate on still-frame photographs but normal structures and pathological lesions within them can be characterised with ease (Fig. 1.7).

Characteristics of ultrasound images

Unlike transmission imaging techniques such as X-rays, ultrasound imaging demonstrates depth in addition to either height or width. Structures that are reflective will be seen as echoes nearest the transducer. The reflective image

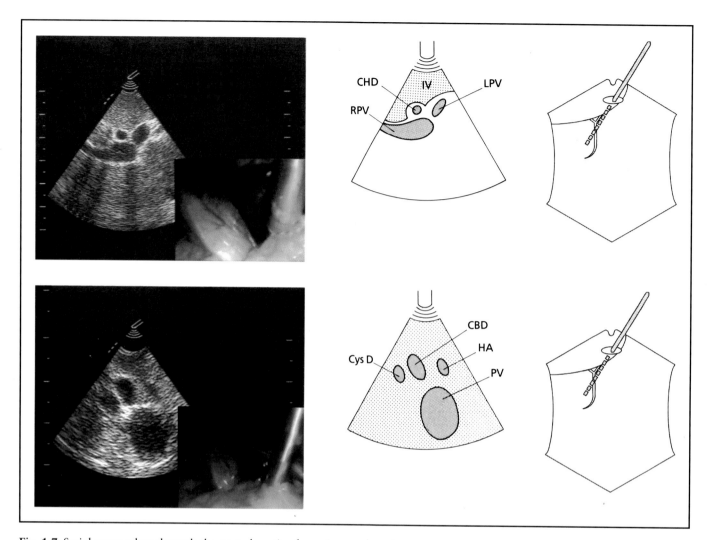

Fig. 1.7 Serial scans taken through the porta hepatis of a patient undergoing laparoscopic cholecystectomy. The sectoral scans show the common bile duct (CBD), the hepatic artery (HA) and the portal vein (PV) as these structures pass through the free edge of the lesser omentum. CHD, common hepatic duct; Cys D, cystic duct; D$_2$, second part of duodenum; GS, gallstone; LPV, left portal vein branch; Panc, pancreas; RPV, right portal vein branch.

is seen in two dimensions as a slice through the tissue, as opposed to the projected (or shadow) image that is obtained by an X-ray (Figs 1.8 and 1.9). The ultrasonographer can orientate the obtained image by the known location of the scanning head and can estimate the size of structures within the tissues from the scan. The surgeon has a considerable advantage over the radiologist in that the obtained image from operative or laparoscopic scanning can be readily related to the structure that is in the surgeon's hand or view.

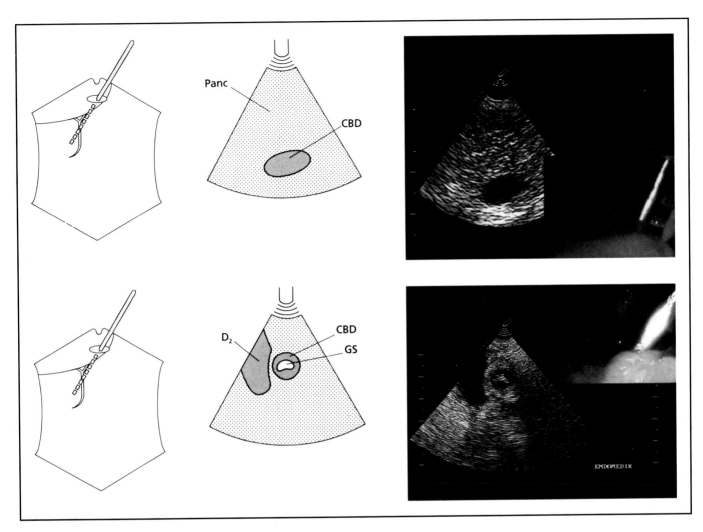

Fig. 1.7 (*Continued*)

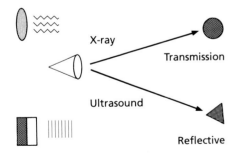

Fig. 1.8 A cone submitted to evaluation by transmission imaging such as X-rays will produce a circular image, whereas the same structure examined by ultrasound will appear as a triangle.

Transducer

The piezoelectric ultrasound transducers produce signals that are affected by the type, shape and size of the crystal and by the frequency of the transmitted ultrasound waves. The beam will remain narrower with higher frequencies, but this can be further maintained by means of focusing. This is achieved by housing an acoustic lens at the transducer surface to refract and converge the sound beams (Fig. 1.10). The focal length is the narrowest cross-section of the beam and objects will be best defined at this distance. Modern real-time ultrasound machines have this facility to focus the beam. It is likely that operative ultrasound probes will be focused on the near field since there is no need to penetrate structures (such as the abdominal wall) which are of little interest to the surgeon. On the other hand, the abdominal

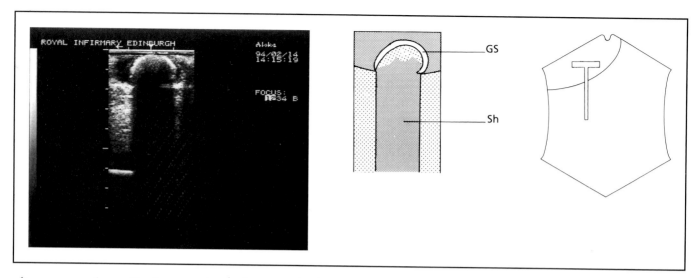

ultrasonographer will often require to focus in the far field to obtain clear images of the abdominal organs.

The cross-section of the ultrasound beam will affect the sharpness of the image because it determines lateral resolution. This is the ability of the ultrasound scan to distinguish the separateness of two reflecting points situated on a plane at right angles to the beam. For two reflective points to be distinguished as two distinct echoes in the same sector scan, they must be separated by at least one beam width. In other words, a narrow beam width produces higher lateral resolution. This differs from axial resolution: the ability to distinguish two points on the axis of the ultrasound beam. This is determined by the frequency of the ultrasound signal. If, for example, two reflective points are located on the same ultrasound beam axis, their echoes cannot be distinguished as two distinct echoes unless the distance between them is greater than the pulse length. Higher frequency permits the use of a shorter pulse length and, hence, ultrasound probes of higher frequency can produce images of exceptional quality by providing greater axial resolution.

These factors are crucial to the choice of ultrasound probe by the clinician. Where penetration of the tissues is important, a low-frequency probe will be required (e.g. 3.5–5 MHz). Resolution may be compromised as a result and may be as high as 5 mm. When there is no need for extensive penetration of tissues, real-time scanners with ultrasound probes of 7.5–10 MHz will provide lateral and axial resolution of 1 mm or less.

To provide real-time images, the individual frames must have accumu-

Fig. 1.9 An intraoperative ultrasound scan of the gallbladder which contains a gallstone (GS) measuring 2 cm in diameter (the scan is marked at 1 cm intervals). Note the marked posterior acoustic shadowing (Sh) which arises from the inability of the ultrasound waves to pass through this solid structure.

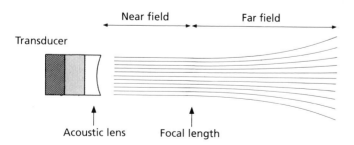

Fig. 1.10 The acoustic lens enables focusing of the ultrasound beam and there is defraction of the ultrasound beam beyond the focal length.

lated maximum information and yet change as rapidly as possible. The higher the rate at which the multiple-pulse echoes are generated, the more restricted the range of depth of penetration. This arises because of the shorter time available for pulses to be transmitted and returned to the transducer.

Both operative and laparoscopic ultrasonography are not subject to the same restrictions that are imposed on abdominal ultrasonography. There is no need for the same tissue penetration, and the high-frequency ultrasound probes will produce better resolution and real-time imaging with rapid pulse repetition rates. The resultant images will be of high quality and provide the clinician with a detailed dynamic investigative tool.

Ultrasound equipment

Real-time B-mode scanning instruments are employed for operative ultrasound imaging. Modern equipment is compact and transportable but it is likely that the surgeon will wish to have a machine available in the operating room and have this dedicated for operative use. The clinician should ensure that the machine can be employed safely in the operating suite and can take the variety of transducers which may be required for specific aspects of his/her operative work. Some of the compact transportable machines can be fitted with abdominal transducers and may be useful in the ward or clinic setting. The surgeon may not wish to be restricted by purchasing a machine that can only take a single dedicated probe thereby compromising subsequent development of the use of ultrasound in the surgeon's clinical practice. Equally, it should be borne in mind that it may be unnecessary to purchase an advanced and expensive item of equipment which will not lend itself readily to use in the operating theatre. We do not see the need to purchase an advanced ultrasound machine costing in excess of £50 000, unless the clinician anticipates sharing its use with radiological colleagues who have a routine requirement for abdominal and Doppler ultrasound imaging. It should also be borne in mind that the more sophisticated the instrument, the more likely the machine will prove difficult to use. Attending theatre staff may experience problems in coping with the complex array of dials and buttons on such a machine.

Transducer probes

It has been our own preference to use linear-array ultrasound probes intraoperatively. The abdominal ultrasonographer prefers to employ a sector ultrasound probe because of the need to maintain good contact with the skin and to access the intra-abdominal organs through a 'window' such as the intercostal rib space (Fig. 1.11). In operative ultrasonography the scan produced by the linear-array transducer will allow the examiner to visualise more clearly the structures near the transducer. Orientation of the anatomy and recognition of abnormalities in the tissues are better appreciated than with sector scanners in this setting.

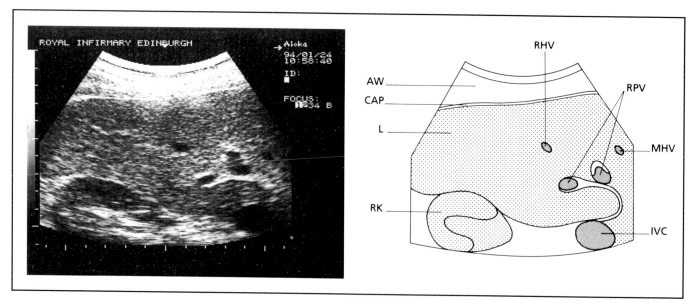

The selection of transducers for specific indications will be covered in the appropriate chapter. However, the linear-array transducers are ideal for examination of the liver, biliary tract, pancreas and kidney since they can be placed flat on the organ of interest and will enable the clinician to build a picture of the anatomy and any tissue abnormalities. The sector scanners are preferred where access is limited and the defined area of interest is small. These are routinely in use in vascular surgery and may be useful in evaluation of the biliary tree or organs in the retroperitoneum or pelvis. Recent advances in the development of laparoscopic sectoral ultrasound probes suggest that these may be more appropriate in the evaluation of the biliary tree and pancreas.

Linear-array transducers are made in either an I-shape or a T-shape (Fig. 1.12) with the connecting cable emerging in line with or at right angles to the transducer head. A side scanning T-shape probe is valuable in examining the liver and the I-shaped probe can be held in the examining surgeon's fingers to gain access to otherwise inaccessible parts of the abdomen at open

Fig. 1.11 Abdominal ultrasound scan taken through the right lower intercostal space with a 3.5 MHz sectoral probe. Note the interference produced by the reflection of ultrasound from the abdominal wall (AW) and liver capsule (CAP). The right hepatic vein (RHV) and right portal vein (RPV) are poorly visualised and the outline of the right kidney (RK) and inferior vena cava (IVC) are seen posteriorly. L, liver parenchyma; MHV, middle hepatic vein.

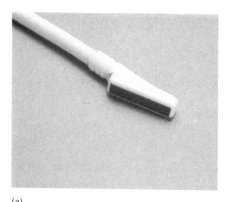

(a)

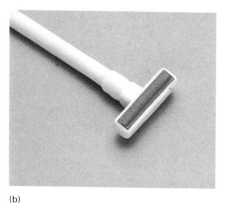

(b)

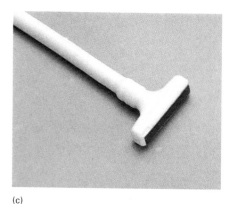

(c)

Fig. 1.12 I-shaped (a) and T-shaped (b–c; side- and end-viewing) linear-array ultrasound probes.

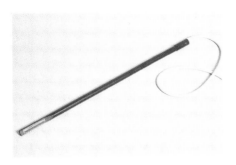

Fig. 1.13 I-shaped linear-array probe used for laparoscopic evaluation.

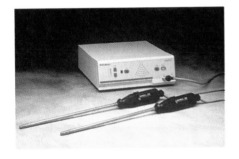

Fig. 1.14 End- and side-viewing sectoral laparoscopic ultrasound probes.

surgery. The I-shape has been embraced in the development of laparoscopic ultrasound probes since these have to be passed through a laparoscopic cannula that has a maximal diameter of 11 mm (Fig. 1.13). Sectoral scanners can be more readily accommodated into these cannulae, but the scan field may be more limited and the surgeon may experience some difficulty in orientation without having the intra-abdominal organ in the examining hand (Fig. 1.14). Some workers have attempted to employ mechanical rotatory probes for use in open and laparoscopic surgery. Such probes may produce high-resolution images, but there is a considerable amount of unnecessary information provided and interpretation of the resultant image is not easy (Fig. 1.15).

Sterilisation

Ultrasound transducers can be prepared for intraoperative use by means of cold gas sterilisation, immersion in a sterilising fluid medium or by employing a disposable plastic sterile cover.

Gas sterilisation with ethylene oxide is the preferred method but is often impractical on the grounds of cost and requirement that the ethylene oxide be allowed to clear by evaporation for several days before the probe is suitable for use. A number of probes would need to be purchased to maintain one ultrasound machine. It should be borne in mind that the connecting cable and the plastic acoustic window of the probe are likely to be damaged if temperatures in excess of 120°F (322 k) are employed in the sterilisation process.

A clean but non-sterile transducer can be placed within a disposable tubular plastic sterile sheet similar to the type that are employed for covering the laparoscopic camera and other similar equipment in the operating theatre. The probe can be threaded, in a sterile manner, into the lumen of the sleeve that is held open by the surgeon or nurse. Approximately 30 ml of methyl cellulose gel should be introduced before the plastic sleeve is threaded over the connecting cable. The cover can be secured over the gel and probe by sterile adhesive tape. The main drawback with this system is the impaired contact between the probe and the organ to be examined. Air bubbles in the

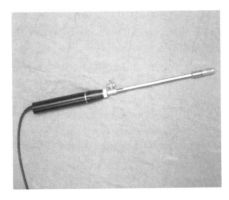

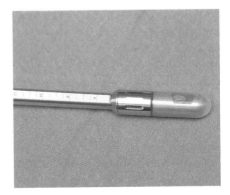

Fig. 1.15 Rotatory mechanical ultrasound probe adapted for laparoscopic use.

gel will produce acoustic shadowing and the plastic sheet itself will reflect some of the ultrasound waves from the transducer. This technique does not readily lend itself to use with laparoscopic ultrasound probes.

The most practical method of sterilising the operative and laparoscopic ultrasound probes is the use of a liquid sterilisation technique. This has the advantage that there is minimal risk of damage to the cable and plastic head. Care must be taken not to immerse the connection to the ultrasound machine since this can be damaged by the corrosive nature of these solutions. We recommend covering this connection with a small plastic bag to prevent inadvertent spillage of the sterilising solution whilst the probe and cable are immersed in the sterilising tray. We use Cidex (glutaraldehyde) and leave the equipment in solution for a minimum of 20 minutes. Before the ultrasound probe is used it should be thoroughly rinsed in sterile water or saline to avoid contact of the sterilising solution with the patient. Other solutions that have been recommended for this type of sterilisation include formalin and Chlorhexidine (Hibitane). Most clinicians will find that liquid sterilisation is the best method for providing easy access to ultrasound probes without the need for purchasing large numbers of probes.

Ultrasound machine

The ultrasound machine has become more sophisticated over the years and comprises a pulse processor, filters, timers, a monitor and alphanumeric keyboard (Fig. 1.16). This equipment produces high-frequency pulses of electric

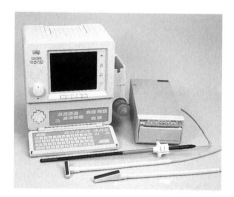
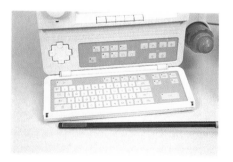
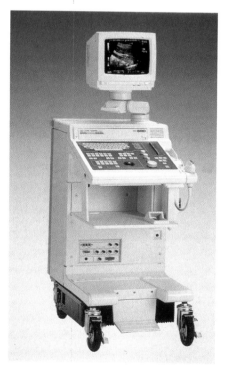

Fig. 1.16 Ultrasound machine used for intraoperative and laparoscopic ultrasonography.

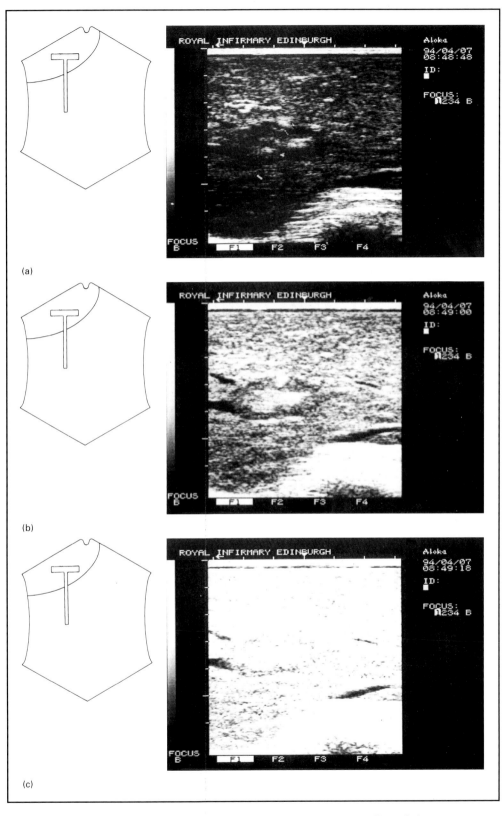

Fig. 1.17 Intraoperative ultrasound scan demonstrating the effect of changes in gain control on the obtained image. With the gain control reduced (a), the obvious metastasis seen in (b) is barely visible. An increase in gain (c) still enables visualisation of the lesion but assessment of the remaining liver is rendered difficult.

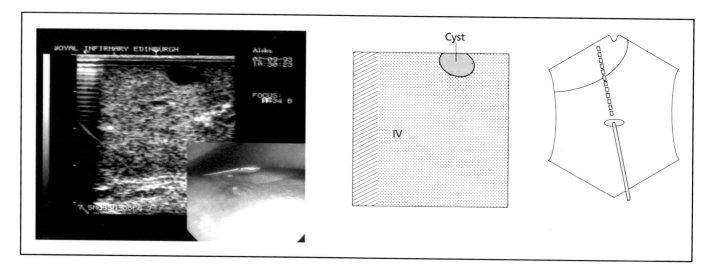

current to the transducer crystal and receives the weaker electric signals produced by reflected ultrasound waves in the transducer crystals. The returned signals are amplified and processed to produce a two-dimensional image. The intensity of the signal on the screen is proportional to the strength of the returning pulses which are displayed as a shade of grey. Smaller portable machines may use less than 20 shades whereas larger more sophisticated equipment will employ as many as 300 shades of grey.

Real-time B-mode ultrasound machines will produce images of various intensities and these indicate the strength of the echoes returning from the tissues. The echogenicity or echoity of the tissues is seen as the ability of the examined tissues to produce echoes and these will be seen on the monitor as various shades of grey. The clinician will need to set the overall or total gain control which will adjust the relative brightness of the image. This adjustment can affect the ability to detect abnormalities in the tissues (Fig. 1.17). Structures that do not reflect ultrasound waves such as a liver cyst would be termed anoechoic or hypoechoic (Fig. 1.18), whereas structures that are highly reflective such as a gallbladder stone (see Fig. 1.9) are termed as hyperechogenic or hyperechoic. Since the examined structures do not produce but merely reflect ultrasound waves, it is more correct to employ the terms echoic, hypoechoic and hyperechoic.

The monitor may be small and compact if it is an integral part of the machine. We have found it useful to display the ultrasound image on a larger screen. For laparoscopic use we employ a digital video mixer (Fig. 1.19) which allows mixing of the laparoscopic camera view at the same time as the ultrasound image is displayed (Figs 1.20 and 1.21).

Permanent records of the ultrasound images can be made either in continuous form with the use of a video recorder or by taking a still photograph. Most ultrasound machines will have the facility to take a camera although it is our own preference to use an electronic recorder which uses heat sensitive paper. This machine can be set in advance, requires little manipulation and can be wired into the video circuit without significant

Fig. 1.18 Laparoscopic ultrasound scan of the liver taken through segment IV demonstrating a hypoechoic lesion which was subsequently confirmed to represent a hepatic cyst. Note the acoustic enhancement of the image which results from the smooth passage of ultrasound waves through the cyst fluid.

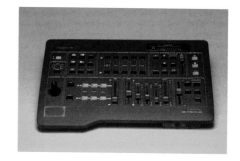

Fig. 1.19 Digital video mixer employed during laparoscopic ultrasonography.

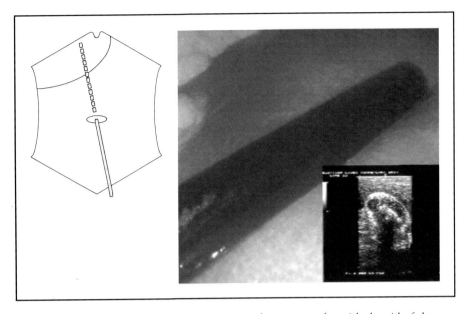

Fig. 1.20 Image obtained during laparoscopic ultrasonography with the aid of the digital video mixer. The ultrasound scan shows a gallbladder full of hyperechoic gallstones.

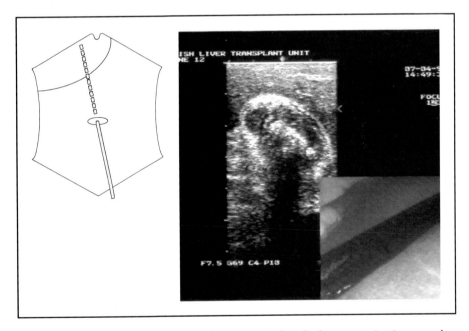

Fig. 1.21 The same image as obtained in Fig. 1.20, but the laparoscopic picture and ultrasound image have been reversed to highlight the position of the ultrasound probe on the liver.

degrading of the image (Fig. 1.22). Sonogram pictures taken from videotape recordings are of inferior quality and it is therefore preferable to make a permanent recording at the time of the initial ultrasound examination.

Operating theatre safety

There is no significant risk to the patient or tissues as a result of the heat generated from diagnostic ultrasound machines. The amount of heat generated from an operative ultrasound probe is almost 5000 times less than that required to produce any harmful biological effect to the tissues.

There are, however, potential dangers in using this form of electrical equipment in the operating theatre environment and all precautions must be taken to prevent the risk of electrical or burn injury to the patient. Tolerance to leakage of current from electrical devices decreases once the skin barrier is removed. The equipment must be submitted to both manufacturer's and standard theatre safety checks similar to that which is undertaken for other theatre equipment.

Operating

The clinician should become familiar with the equipment before embarking on an operative examination and to avoid an unhappy initial experience! It is useful to have a colleague or trained individual available who can deal with the non-sterile ultrasound machine whilst the surgeon is preoccupied with the transducer probe.

Whereas the radiologist requires a coupling gel to produce good quality images this is not the case in operative ultrasonography. The probe can generally be placed in direct contact with the organ to be examined without the need for gel. If good contact cannot be obtained in this way, such as is required in direct assessment of the biliary tree, it is suggested that the surgeon instil some sterile physiological saline into the abdomen. The small microbubbles of air do not generally produce significant interference to the ultrasound images.

With all ultrasound probes there is a loss of image immediately next to the surface of the transducer head, although with the higher frequency probes this loss is unlikely to prove a significant handicap to the surgeon during examination of solid organs. Superficial lesions on the liver, for example, are likely to be visible to the naked eye even if they cannot be readily imaged on the ultrasound scan. The instillation of saline may be of value during intraoperative and laparoscopic ultrasonography and some authors have suggested the use of a saline filled pouch at open surgery to prevent the loss of field immediately beneath the probe.

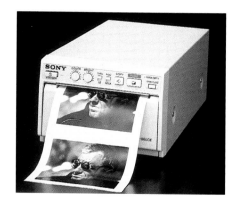

Fig. 1.22 Camera used for documenting ultrasound images on heat sensitive paper.

2: The Gallbladder and Bile Ducts

Introduction

Intraoperative evaluation of the extrahepatic biliary tree by ultrasound was a technique first proposed in the 1960s by workers in the United Kingdom [1] and in the United States [2]. The early A-mode scanners available at that time produced uni-dimensional images which, although capable of detecting gallstones, could be difficult to interpret. B-mode intraoperative ultrasound systems later became available in the 1980s and provided easily recognisable, high-resolution, two-dimensional images of the underlying tissues, and its utility in detecting choledocholithiasis was enthusiastically reported in the English literature by Lane and Glazer [3] and in the American literature by Sigel *et al.* [4,5]. However, only a few surgeons championed its routine use during open biliary tract surgery [6,7], reporting intraoperative ultrasound to be at least as accurate as operative cholangiography in the detection of choledocholithiasis. It was evident that operative cholangiography could be undertaken at open cholecystectomy with relative ease and that the anatomy of the biliary tree could be better defined by cholangiography than by intraoperative ultrasonography.

The development of laparoscopic cholecystectomy has renewed interest in the use of contact ultrasound at operation. There remains controversy regarding the need for intraoperative cholangiography during laparoscopic cholecystectomy, and although success rates exceeding 90% can be expected with experience [8,9], many laparoscopic surgeons continue to pursue a policy of selective cholangiography. Furthermore, some have abandoned the procedure in favour of preoperative endoscopic retrograde or intravenous cholangiography. The development of high-resolution contact ultrasound probes that may be used during laparoscopy provides an alternative means of assessing the biliary tract for the presence of gallstones and in the evaluation of bile duct neoplasms.

This chapter will provide detailed descriptions of the technique of intraoperative and laparoscopic ultrasonography, highlighting their role in the detection of calculi in the extrahepatic biliary tree. The use of ultrasound in the evaluation of malignant obstruction of the biliary tract will be more fully discussed in Chapter 4, but its use in the assessment of high bile duct obstruction will be covered in the appropriate sections below.

Anatomy (Figs 2.1 and 2.2)

The biliary tree can be conveniently separated into three parts: (i) the gallbladder; (ii) the intrahepatic ducts; and (iii) the extrahepatic biliary tree. The gallbladder is situated on the undersurface of the right lobe of the liver

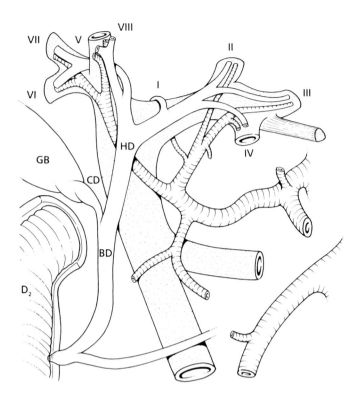

Fig. 2.1 The biliary tree. The segmental branches (I–VIII) drain the right and left hemilivers to form the right and left hepatic ducts. The cystic (CD) and common hepatic (HD) ducts join to form the common bile duct (BD). The right hepatic artery is shown running between the portal vein and the HD. D₂, second part of duodenum; GB, gallbladder.

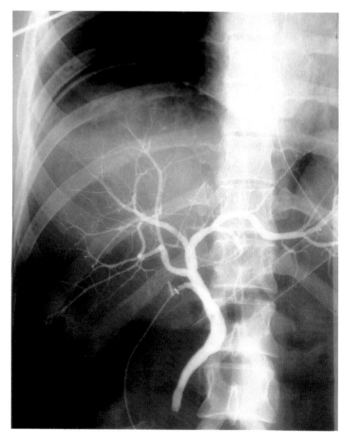

Fig. 2.2 An operative cholangiogram taken during a laparoscopic cholecystectomy. Note the low entry of the posterior sectoral duct below the confluence of the left hepatic and anterior sectoral duct. There is no flow of contrast into the duodenum and at least two small stones are seen in the cystic and common bile ducts.

between segments IV and V. The middle hepatic vein runs in a plane that passes through the gallbladder bed to the left side of the inferior vena cava and which separates the liver into its right and left halves. The cystic duct passes from the spiral valves of Hartmann's pouch to join the common hepatic duct at a variable position in the lesser omentum.

The right and left hepatic ducts are formed from the segmental ducts within the liver. The ducts from segments VI and VII join as the posterior sectoral duct. The segmental ducts V and VIII link to form the anterior sectoral duct whose confluence with the posterior duct forms the right hepatic duct. This latter confluence is usually intrahepatic, but there is considerable variation in the level of this confluence and indeed variation in the precise configuration of the segmental ducts. These ducts are closely related to the segmental branches of the hepatic artery and portal vein and are enveloped by Glisson's capsule as these structures pass into the liver substance. This dense capsule enables the ultrasonographer to differentiate readily the portal structures from the hepatic veins that have no such hyperechoic wall (Fig. 2.3).

The ducts from segments II and III (left hepatic lobe) join with that of segment IV (quadrate lobe) in the umbilical fissure of the liver. The obliter-

Fig. 2.3 Intraoperative ultrasound scan of the liver showing the middle hepatic vein (MHV) and the portal pedicle containing the right (RHD) and left (LHD) hepatic ducts, the proper hepatic artery (PHA) and the anterior sectoral hepatic artery (ASHA). Note the hyperechoic image cast by the dense capsule around the structures at the porta hepatis and the absence of a defined wall to the hepatic vein. LPV, left portal vein.

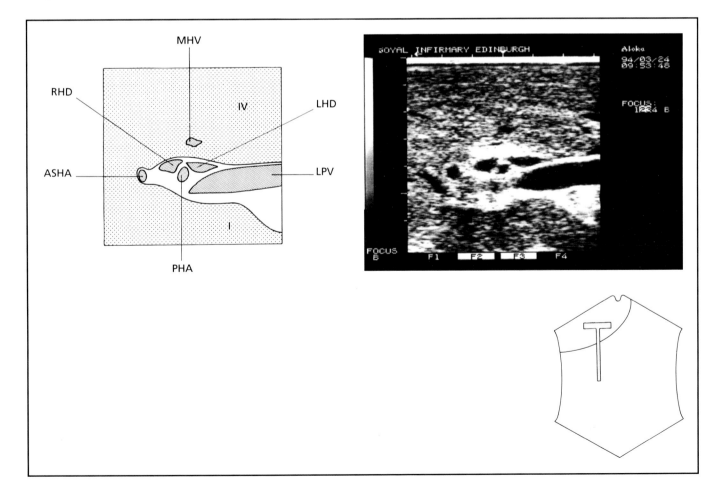

ated umbilical vein passes in the free edge of the falciform ligament to fuse
with the sheath of the portal pedicle at this point. The segmental ducts form
the left hepatic duct, which runs an extrahepatic course at the base of segment IV before its confluence with the right duct at the hilus of the liver. The
duct(s) from segment I (caudate lobe) are variable in position but generally
join the left hepatic duct before or at its confluence with the left duct.

The bile ducts lie anterior to the branches of the portal vein and hepatic
artery within the liver substance, but the relative position of the ducts and
the arterial branches in the porta hepatis are more variable. The right branch
of the hepatic artery may, for example, pass in front of the common hepatic
duct or course between it and the portal vein (see Fig. 2.1). Alternatively, the
right hepatic artery may arise from the superior mesenteric artery or directly
from the aorta, and pass behind the portal vein to run along its lateral border in the free edge of the lesser omentum (Fig. 2.4).

The relationship of the supraduodenal and infraduodenal portions of the
common bile duct to other structures is more constant. The duct passes behind the first part of the duodenum anterior to the superior pancreaticoduodenal artery to join the pancreatic duct within the head of the
pancreas. The presence of a common channel is variable as the ducts open
into the second part of the duodenum at the ampulla of Vater.

Ultrasound examination of the normal biliary tree

The biliary tree can be evaluated with either a linear-array or sectoral probe.
It is generally easier for the beginner to employ a linear-array ultrasound
probe which can be placed flat on the liver to examine the intrahepatic biliary
tree and the gallbladder. In this way, the surgeon can readily identify the
various anatomical landmarks and establish their relationships. It is our own
practice to employ a T-shaped 5 or 7.5 MHz linear-array probe at open
surgery and the evaluation of the biliary tree using this instrument will be
described.

Fig. 2.4 Laparoscopic ultrasound scan
with the probe placed over the gastric
antrum (insert) showing an accessory
right hepatic artery (RHA) arising from
the superior mesenteric artery to pass
behind the portal vein (PV). The distal
common bile duct (CBD) is seen
traversing the head of the pancreas (HP).

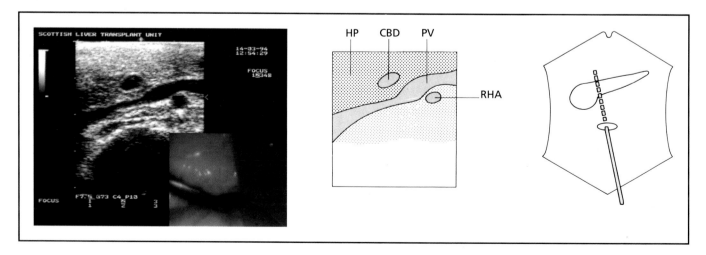

Intraoperative ultrasonography

The gallbladder

At laparotomy, the gallbladder can be easily examined and it is helpful for the inexperienced ultrasonographer to start at this site. The ultrasound probe is placed on the anterior surface of segments IV and V with the probe orientated transversely. The gallbladder is easily recognised by its echogenic wall and hypoechoic bile within its lumen (Fig. 2.5). Since the ultrasound waves pass easily through the bile there may be prominent acoustic enhancement posteriorly (see Chapter 1).

A layer of sludge or hyperechoic debris may be observed on the posterior gallbladder wall, and gentle agitation may produce a small cloud of particles within the gallbladder. These can be differentiated from small gallbladder calculi which will settle to the gallbladder floor more rapidly, and which typically appear densely hyperechoic with posterior shadowing (Fig. 2.5). The gallbladder wall appears hyperechoic, and in the normal individual will be thin walled, measure less than 3 mm in thickness and exhibits three distinct echo-layers. Mucosal projections may be evident and will be most prominent as the probe is displaced to examine Hartmann's pouch. It may be possible to trace the cystic duct to its confluence with the common hepatic duct by carefully displacing the probe inferiorly. The cystic duct may be more readily recognised by placing the probe sagittally on segment IV to identify the common hepatic and bile ducts in the first instance (Fig. 2.6).

The intrahepatic ducts

The intrahepatic ducts may be examined with the transducer placed on the liver surface. The walls of the bile ducts appear hyperechoic due to the investing fascial sheath derived from the liver capsule, and they lie alongside the corresponding branch of the hepatic artery and portal vein within the liver substance. A more detailed description of their intrahepatic course will be given in Chapter 3. They may be traced to the porta hepatis with the

Fig. 2.5 Intraoperative sonogram obtained with a linear-array probe placed over the quadrate lobe (segment IV) of the liver. A thick-walled oedematous gallbladder (GB) containing a 1 cm calculus (GS) is demonstrated. The sonogram is orientated in a sagittal plane, and loss of transducer contact is noted to the left of the image. The inferior vena cava (IVC) is barely visible behind the caudate lobe (segment I).

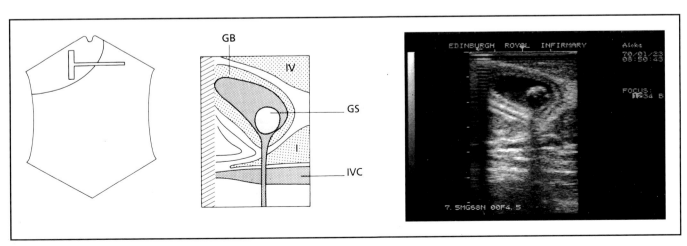

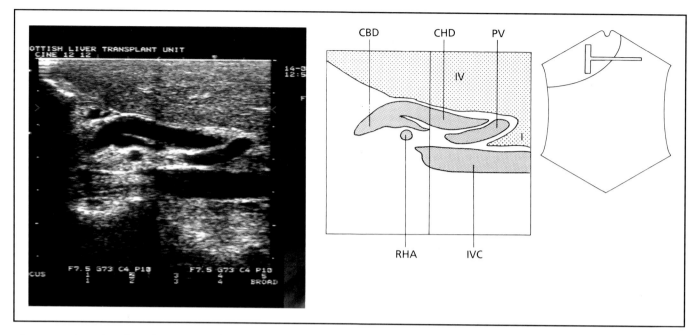

ultrasound probe placed transversely on the anterior surface of segment IV (see Fig. 2.3). It is necessary to gently incline the probe upwards and downwards to best locate the segmental and sectoral ducts. The ultrasonographer should be able to identify the common hepatic duct anterior to the portal vein and so trace the smaller ducts into the liver from the porta hepatis.

In the normal individual it is often quite difficult to identify a non-dilated intrahepatic duct which, if seen, is the same size as the pulsatile intrahepatic branches of the hepatic artery. Failure to visualise the intrahepatic ducts using a 5–7.5 MHz contact ultrasound probe usually indicates the absence of obvious pathology causing dilatation of the proximal biliary tree.

The extrahepatic biliary tree

The extrahepatic biliary tree may be examined in several planes using a linear-array transducer which may be positioned in a predominantly transverse or sagittal orientation. It is advisable that the surgeon avoids unnecessary dissection and mobilisation of the liver before the initial ultrasound examination as the introduction of air in the subhepatic space may produce considerable artefact, preventing adequate visualisation of the duct system and diminishing the advantages of contact ultrasound. The examination commences with the probe placed in a transverse position on the anterior surface of segment IV. The extrahepatic course of the left hepatic duct is located anterior to the left branch of the portal vein, and the various segmental ducts may be located as they lie in contact with the segmental branches of the portal vein (Fig. 2.7). The obliterated umbilical vein often appears as a bright hyperechoic lesion, and this appearance must not be confused with an intrahepatic calculus which would typically be associated with some proximal duct dilatation.

Fig. 2.6 Intraoperative sonogram obtained with a linear-array transducer placed on the quadrate lobe of the liver (segment IV) in a plane passing through the long axis of the hepatic pedicle. The cystic duct confluence with the common hepatic duct (CHD) is posterior. An accessory right hepatic artery (RHA) passes dorsal to these structures. The caudate lobe (segment I) is seen separating the portal vein (PV) and inferior vena cava (IVC) like a wedge. CBD, common bile duct.

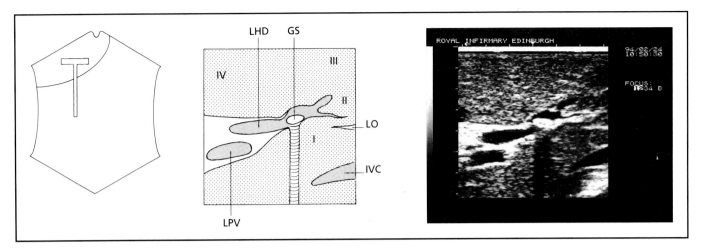

Fig. 2.7 Intraoperative sonogram obtained with the transducer placed transversely on the left hemiliver. A gallstone (GS) is observed in the left hepatic duct (LHD). The segmental ducts to II and III can be seen anterior to the fascial insertion of the lesser omentum (LO). IVC, inferior vena cava; LPV, left portal vein.

The confluence of the left and right duct systems can be identified anterior to the bifurcation of the portal vein at the liver hilum (Fig. 2.8). The right hepatic artery usually passes between these two structures. The high velocity, low pressure flow of blood within the portal vein is usually visible, and this structure is easily differentiated from the hepatic artery, which is pulsatile, and the vena cava, which conveys the pulsations of the cardiac cycle from the right atrium. The diameter of the common duct is variable and opinions vary as to its normal range. However, it is reasonable to regard the duct as normally measuring less than or equal to 8 mm in the elderly patient, and less than or equal to 6 mm in a younger individual. It is convenient to measure the maximum diameter of the common hepatic duct in the porta hepatis using the electronic calipers which are a feature of most intraoperative ultrasound scanners (Fig. 2.8(d)). Care should be taken not to compress the duct by excessive down pressure from the probe.

It may be possible for the clinician to examine the entire supraduodenal portion of the bile duct without having to displace the probe from the quadrate lobe of the liver. If this is not possible, the transducer should be moved directly onto the free edge of the lesser omentum. Some loss of the near-field image directly beneath the transducer may be unavoidable (see Chapter 1), and it may be useful to instill saline into the subhepatic space, or to employ a saline filled stand-off, to obtain satisfactory images of the hilar structures. The common hepatic duct lies anterolateral to the portal vein within the free edge of the lesser omentum. The right hepatic artery can usually be identified passing behind the common hepatic duct as it supplies the right liver.

The cystic duct is generally coursing behind the hepatic duct before it joins this structure to form the common bile duct (see Fig. 2.6). However, the level of this confluence is variable and the cystic duct may join the common hepatic duct on any side. The common bile duct runs behind the first part of the duodenum, and follows a divergent lateral course away from the portal vein, passing behind or through the head of the pancreas to join the pancreatic duct at the duodenal papilla. The gastroduodenal artery passes inferiorly with the common bile duct before it gives rise to the superior

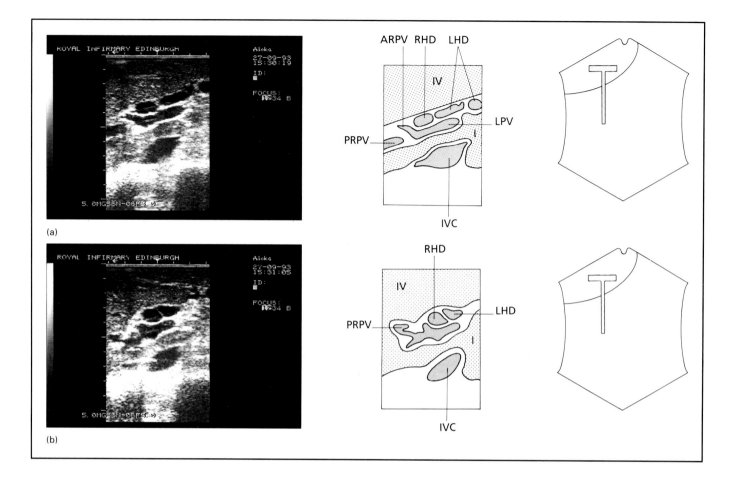

pancreaticoduodenal artery whose relationship with the duct is variable. There may be some interference from gas within the duodenum, and the ultrasonographer may be required to displace the duodenal contents by compression with the probe to improve the quality of the image.

The intrapancreatic portion of the bile duct is best seen with the ultrasound probe placed over the head of the pancreas. The pancreatic duct, which normally measures less than or equal to 3 mm in diameter, may be identified passing over the portal vein, through the pancreatic neck and into a convergent lateral course through the pancreatic head to meet the distal common bile duct (Fig. 2.9).

When the extrahepatic biliary tree is examined using a linear-array intraoperative ultrasound probe orientated in a sagittal plane, the transducer will inevitably lose contact with the surface of the liver as it is displaced inferiorly (see Figs 2.5 and 2.6), and it should be moved directly into parallel contact with the structures passing within the hepatoduodenal ligament. In this way, the tubular structures of the hepatic pedicle are imaged in a predominantly longitudinal axis (Fig. 2.9). A detailed description of the images so obtained will accompany the account of laparoscopic ultrasonography of the bile duct employing a linear-array probe.

Fig. 2.8 Transverse intraoperative sonogram through the porta hepatis with linear-array transducer placed on segment IV. (a) A tortuous dilated left (LHD) and right (RHD) hepatic duct can be seen anterior to the trifurcation of the left portal vein (LPV) and the anterior (ARPV) and posterior (PRPV) sectoral divisions of the right portal vein. (b) The transducer has been displaced inferiorly to show the confluence of the RHD and LHD anterior to the portal trunk and its right posterior branch (PRPV).

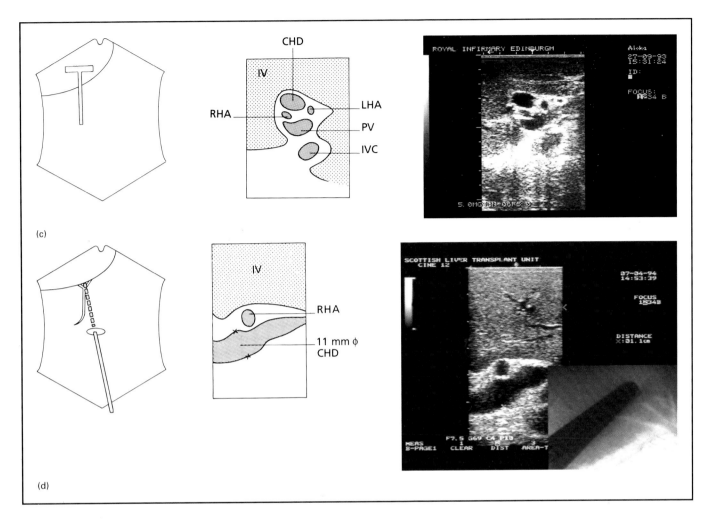

Fig. 2.8 (*Continued*) (c) The dilated common hepatic duct (CHD), which measures 12 mm in diameter, lies anterior to the main portal vein (PV). The right (RHA) and left (LHA) hepatic arteries pass between. The inferior vena cava (IVC) is seen posteriorly.
(d) Laparoscopic sonogram demonstrating a longitudinal cut through the CHD. The maximum diameter of the CHD has been measured as 11 mm using the electronic calipers. Note the RHA passing anterior to the duct.

Laparoscopic ultrasonography

The technique of laparoscopic ultrasonography for examination of the biliary tree during laparoscopic cholecystectomy is based on that of intraoperative ultrasonography at open operation. Access to the peritoneal cavity is attained via 10/11 mm ports which are placed at the umbilical and subxiphoid sites according to the usual 'four-port' convention. Disposable cannulae are preferable to reusable metal ports, as the screening surface and crystals of the transducer are vulnerable to damage from metal trumpet valves. Dissection of the gallbladder pedicle is best avoided at the outset of the procedure as the presence of gas in the tissue spaces may interfere with subsequent imaging of the structures in this area. The examination technique for both linear-array and mechanical sectoral probes will be described since fundamental differences exist between the two.

Laparoscopic ultrasound examination using a linear-array probe

Laparoscopic ultrasonography of the biliary tree during laparoscopic

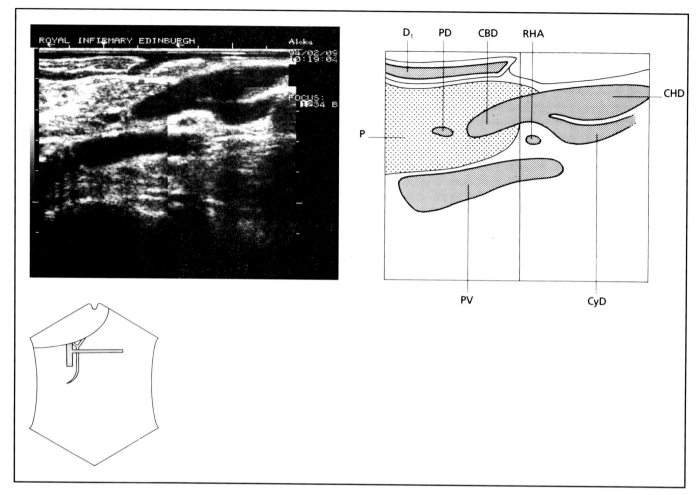

cholecystectomy may be performed with the probe operated from either the umbilical or subxiphoid port. This permits the generation of images in a variety of planes. Whilst both approaches may be required in cases where difficulty is encountered in imaging the entire duct system, the technique favoured to perform the initial screening of the bile ducts varies between surgeons. We prefer to use the probe via the umbilical port, and so obtain longitudinal images of the hilar structures in a predominantly oblique–sagittal scanning plane. The probe may later be inserted through the subxiphoid port, and with the side-viewing linear-array transducer placed in near-vertical apposition with the free edge of the hepatoduodenal ligament, scanning in a transverse direction may be performed to produce cross-sectional images of the hilar structures (Fig. 2.10).

The examination commences with the laparoscopic ultrasound probe inserted via the umbilical port and placed under direct laparoscopic visualisation on the diaphragmatic surface of segments IV (quadrate lobe) and V. This will enable the surgeon to visualise the gallbladder at the outset of the examination and so allow the size and number of any gallstones present to be evaluated along with the size of the gallbladder itself, and the thickness of its wall. The ultrasound probe is swept slowly over the right hemiliver. Rotation of the probe to the patient's right side will allow the surgeon to exam-

Fig. 2.9 Intraoperative sonogram obtained with the linear-array transducer placed sagittally in the long axis of the free edge of the lesser omentum, and over the first part of the duodenum (D_1) and pancreatic head (P). A low, posterior cystic duct (CyD) insertion with the common hepatic duct (CHD) is seen at the upper border of the pancreas. The right hepatic artery (RHA) passes between the common bile duct (CBD) and the portal vein (PV) at this level. The pancreatic duct (PD) is visible in the gland.

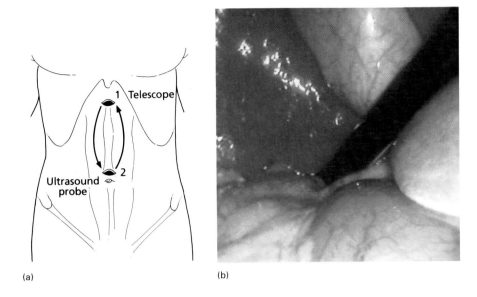

Fig. 2.10 (a) Diagrammatic representation of the position of the ports, telescope (1) and laparoscopic ultrasound probe (2) during evaluation of the biliary tree. (b) Position of the laparoscopic ultrasound probe is perpendicular to the hepatoduodenal ligament having been inserted via a subxiphoid port.

(a)   (b)

ine the right hemiliver, whilst rotation anticlockwise to the left brings the structures at the porta hepatis into view. It may be possible to follow Hartmann's pouch and the cystic duct to the latter's confluence with the hepatic duct.

The bifurcation of the portal vein and hepatic artery are examined through subtle rotatory movements of the probe. It may not be possible for the surgeon at the outset of the examination to readily identify smaller structures, but orientation is best achieved by recognition of the portal vein as the key landmark, which is separated from the inferior vena cava by the caudate lobe of the liver (segment I) (Fig. 2.11). As described above, laminar blood flow is usually visible within the portal vein. In contrast, the hepatic artery is pulsatile and lies anteromedially, whilst the common hepatic duct lies anterolateral to these structures in the free edge of the hepatoduodenal ligament.

The anterior and posterior sectoral divisions of the right branch of the portal vein can be followed out into the right liver, although the associated ducts may not be readily visible unless these are dilated. They, and their corresponding arterial branches, lie anterior to the portal vein branches. The left duct system may be traced through its extrahepatic course as it drains the left liver (Fig. 2.11).

Once as much of the biliary tree as possible has been assessed using the liver as an 'acoustic window', the probe is moved directly onto the porta hepatis and the transducer withdrawn over the first part of the duodenum and the head of the pancreas, to enable the distal common bile duct to be examined (see Fig. 2.4). Care must be taken not to tear any adhesions from the liver or cause trauma to the structures in this area. The instillation of physiological saline into the abdominal cavity may be useful to optimise acoustic contact and minimise probe down pressure which might compress the duct. It is useful to reference the visualised structures to the easily recognisable portal vein. Rotation of the probe clockwise to the patient's right

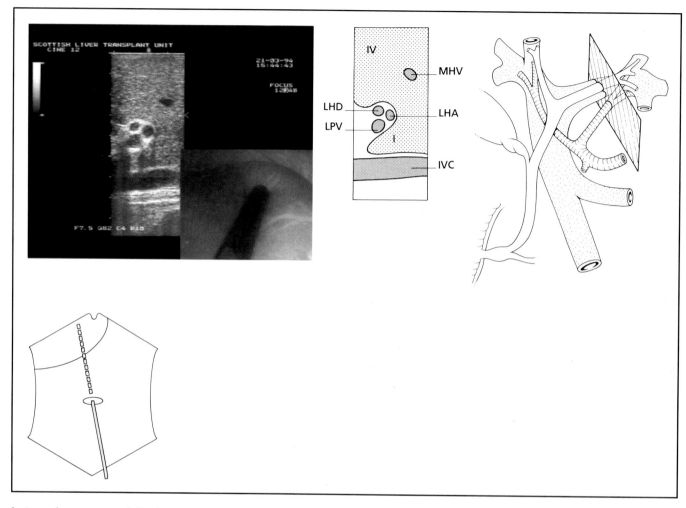

brings the common bile duct into view as it passes from the free edge of the hepatoduodenal ligament behind the first part of the duodenum to traverse the head of the pancreas (see Fig. 2.4). The duodenal wall is identifiable by visible peristalsis and exhibits five distinct echo-layers in continuity with the gastric antrum. Luminal gas may cause acoustic interference and image degradation. This may be minimised by gently compressing the duodenum with the probe, so displacing the underlying gas. The common duct is examined in its oblique distal course through the pancreatic head by gradual rotation of the probe to the right until the duct terminates at the ampulla, marked by the appearance of folds of duodenal mucosa. This part of the laparoscopic ultrasound examination of the biliary tree may be the most difficult if the duct is small or collapsed, or if interference from duodenal gas is encountered. Some authors prefer to position the transducer against the lateral duodenal wall so as to scan medially in a coronal plane, thus obtaining a foreshortened image of the distal common duct [10]. Another source of difficulty may occasionally be encountered in applying the probe to the liver or hepatic pedicle if there is a wide angle of impact between the probe and these structures (Fig. 2.12). This problem may arise in slim patients with a lax abdominal wall in whom the umbilical port site is too near the scanning area, and may be overcome by complete or partial desufflation of the

Fig. 2.11 Sagittally orientated sonogram obtained at laparoscopy with linear-array probe positioned over the left hemiliver. The left portal pedicle is seen in cross-section lying anterior to the caudate lobe (I) and the inferior vena cava (IVC). It comprises the left hepatic duct (LHD), the left hepatic artery (LHA) and the left portal vein (LPV). The accompanying diagram shows the position of the ultrasound probe. MHV, middle hepatic vein.

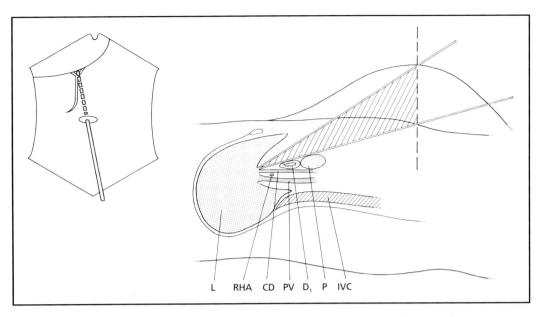

Fig. 2.12 Diagram illustrating the acute angle that may arise between the laparoscopic ultrasound probe and the hepatoduodenal ligament (L) in the slim patient with a lax abdominal wall. Deflation of the peritoneal cavity may improve the contact between probe and porta hepatis (hatched lines). CD, cystic duct; D_1, first part of the duodenum; IVC, inferior vena cava; P, pancreas; PV, portal vein; RHA, right hepatic artery.

Fig. 2.13 Laparoscopic ultrasound examination of the porta hepatis with the linear-array laparoscopic ultrasound probe inserted through the subxiphoid port. The transducer has been placed alongside the free edge of the hepatoduodenal ligament and saline has been instilled to improve acoustic coupling. Note the 'Mickey Mouse' appearance of the common bile duct (CHD), hepatic artery proper (HA) and portal vein (PV) seen in transverse section.

pneumoperitoneum. However, it may be necessary to replace the probe via the subxiphoid port in order to obtain a different perspective and improve image quality if scanning via the umbilical port is unsatisfactory (see Figs 2.10 and 2.13).

As for any ultrasound examination, it is important that the surgeon should avoid rapid movements of the probe. This dynamic investigation is best performed by smooth gentle displacement of the probe with subtle rotational movements. Much tactile feedback is lost at laparoscopy, upon which the surgeon relies at open operation for assessment of the structures at the porta

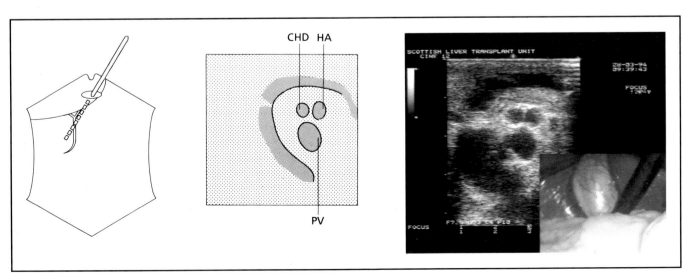

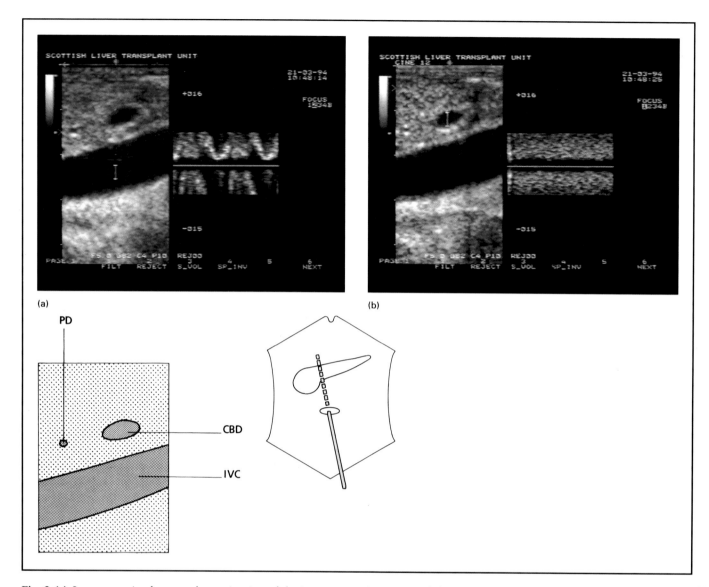

Fig. 2.14 Laparoscopic ultrasound examination of the intrapancreatic common bile duct (CBD). (a) The inferior vena cava (IVC) is readily identified by its characteristic Doppler waveform. (b) The cursor is placed on the CBD which has no detectable flow within it (note the flat Doppler signal). The pancreatic duct (PD) is also visible within the head of the pancreas.

hepatis. Recognition of these structures by laparoscopic ultrasonography may be enhanced if a Doppler flow sampling facility is incorporated with the scanner. This facilitates the rapid detection and characterisation of blood flow within the hilar structures, allowing prompt identification of the hepatic artery, portal vein, inferior vena cava and ductal structures, which may be useful in cases of doubt (Fig. 2.14).

Laparoscopic ultrasound examination using a sector-scanning probe

A variety of mechanical sector-scanning transducers have been evaluated during laparoscopic ultrasonography, with sectoral angles ranging from

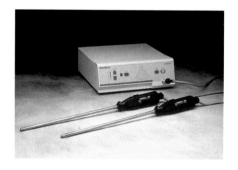

Fig. 2.15 The prototype Endomedix LaparoScan laparoscopic ultrasound system consists of forward- (U750F) and oblique-viewing (U750S) single-crystal 90° sector-scanning transducers at the tip of the rigid probe shaft. The probes are connected to a small electronic scanning machine (U2000).

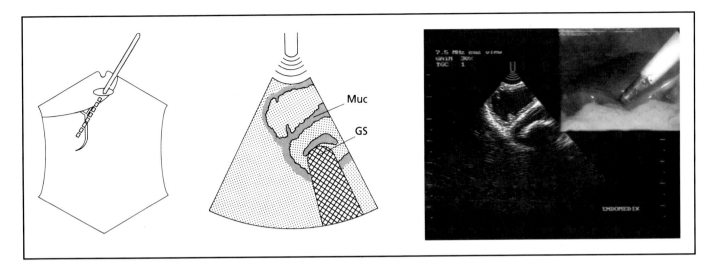

Fig. 2.16 Laparoscopic sonogram taken with a forward-viewing 90° sectoral-scanning probe placed over segment IV demonstrating the gallbladder, which is sigmoid shaped, with a calculus (GS) in Hartmann's pouch. The separate layers of the gallbladder wall are visible. Muc, mucosa.

Fig. 2.17 Laparoscopic sonogram obtained with the oblique-viewing 90° sector-scanning probe placed over segment IV. The common hepatic duct (CHD) and portal vein (PV) are demonstrated in cross-section.

60° to 360°. More recently, convex array or curvilinear-array laparoscopic ultrasound probes have become available, which combine the features of mechanical sectoral scanners and linear-array transducers, to give a trapezoid-shaped sonogram [11,12]. We have evaluated a mechanical sector-scanning probe equipped with a single 4.5 mm diameter crystal, oscillating about a pivot, to generate a 90° sector field of view. Two probes were available and designed for both forward and oblique viewing (Figs 2.15–2.17). Rotation of the probe shaft produced a range of scanning 'cuts' between transverse and sagittal planes, and the entire examination could be performed via a 10/11 mm subxiphoid port.

With the probe tip placed upon the right lobe of the liver, the gallbladder and hilar structures are examined as described above. Optimal scanning of the extrahepatic biliary tree is achieved by moving the tip of the probe from the liver into direct contact with the free edge of the lesser omentum, retracting the gallbladder superiorly with grasping forceps via a lateral port as required. In contrast to the technique employed for the linear-array probe, it is our preference to evaluate the hepatoduodenal ligament in a predominantly transverse plane (Fig. 2.18(a,b)). In this way, the duct can be kept in constant view and is traced along its entire length. Care must be taken to

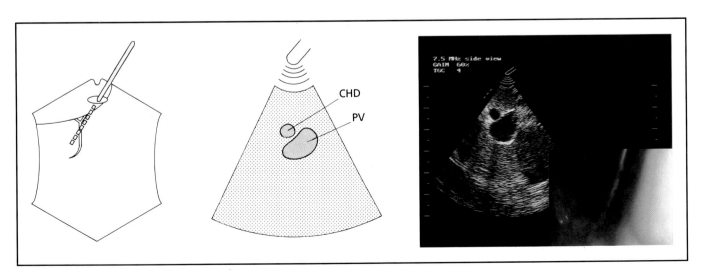

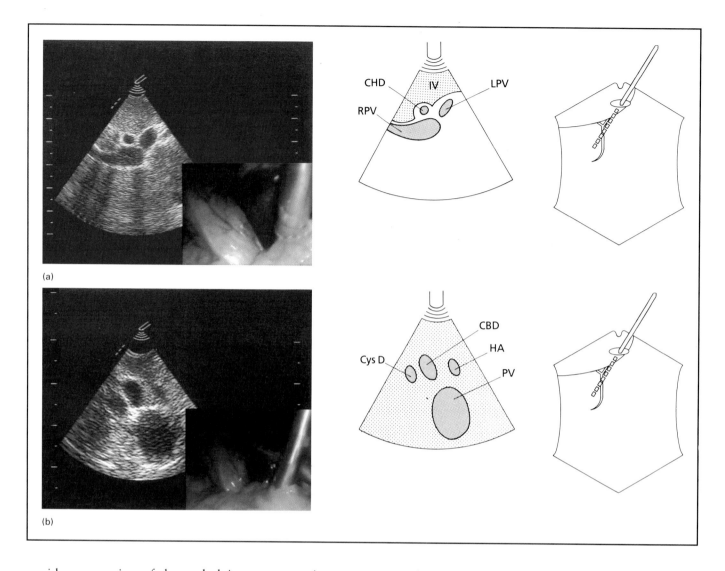

avoid compression of the underlying structures in an attempt to improve probe contact. Such manoeuvres are counter-productive if they cause luminal obliteration and cause the ultrasonographer to miss even diseased bile ducts. Once the anatomy of the hepatic pedicle has been identified, the common duct is traced distally through the head of the pancreas to its termination with the pancreatic duct at the papilla of Vater (Fig. 2.18(c,d)).

The radially orientated cuts obtained with the sector-scanning probe can be somewhat disorientating to the surgeon early in his/her experience. The smaller cross-sectional area of the transducer screening surface can result in amplified shifts in the image following only subtle movements of the probe handpiece. By contrast, the rectilinear sonograms obtained from flat, side-viewing linear-arrary transducers are more stable and easier to interpret. However, once the technique is mastered, excellent images of the common bile duct can be obtained through to the papilla in the majority of patients using a mechanical sector-scanning probe.

Fig. 2.18 A sequence of laparoscopic sonograms of the extrahepatic biliary tree obtained with the oblique-viewing 90° sector-scanning probe inserted through the subxiphoid port. (a) The probe has been placed on segment IV and the common hepatic duct (CHD) is seen anterior to the bifurcation of the portal vein. (b) Cross-sectional image of the common bile duct (CBD), cystic duct (CysD), hepatic artery (HA) and the portal vein (PV) within the free edge of the hepatoduodenal ligament ('Mickey Mouse' view).

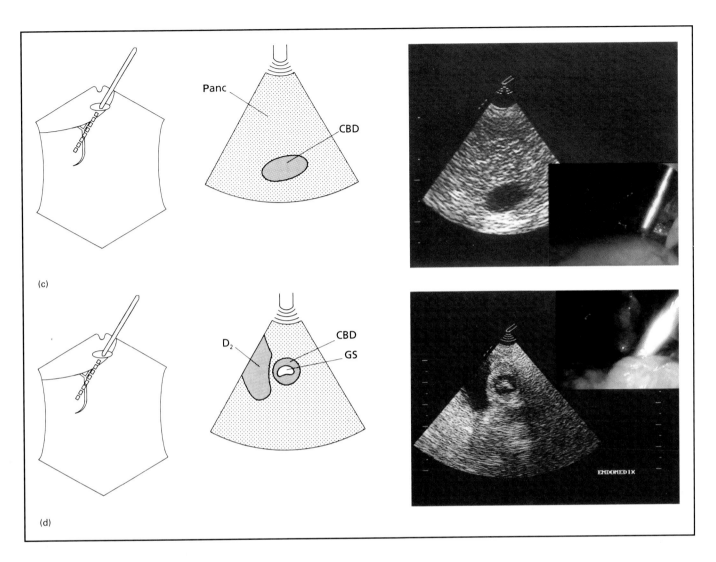

Fig. 2.18 (*Continued*) (c) The distal CBD has been traced through its intrapancreatic portion (Panc). (d) An unsuspected finding of an impacted calculus (GS) in the distal CBD proximal to the ampulla. D₂, lumen of second part of duodenum; LPV, left portal vein; RPV, right portal vein.

Cholelithiasis

The diagnosis of gallstones will usually have been made preoperatively, but it is useful to dwell on the features of gallbladder pathology since ultrasound examination of the gallbladder is a good form of training for the surgeon undertaking intraoperative or laparoscopic ultrasonography. Conversely, it is important to confirm or exclude the presence of gallstones if the diagnosis of cholelithiasis has not been made preoperatively, e.g. in the patient undergoing urgent surgery for the complications of acute pancreatitis (Fig. 2.19).

In the patient with gallstones, the ultrasound examination may reveal a distended gallbladder filled with anechoic bile. The gallstone will invariably be situated posteriorly and will be seen as a crescentic hyperechoic image associated with posterior acoustic shadowing. The posterior aspect of the stone will not be evident since the ultrasound waves are completely reflected by the calculus (see Figs 2.19–2.21). The size of the stone(s) can be documented, and sludge or microcalculi will be seen as a layer of hyperechoic material settled on the posterior wall of the gallbladder (Fig. 2.20). The gallbladder wall thickness may be assessed, and the signs of mural inflam-

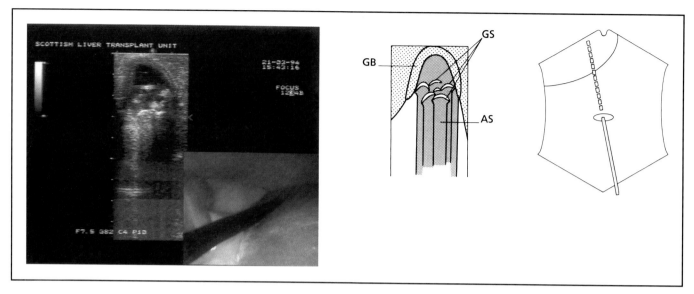

Fig. 2.19 Laparoscopic sonogram demonstrating multiple small gallstones (GS) within a thick-walled gallbladder (GB) in a patient undergoing laparoscopic cholecystectomy following an episode of gallstone related acute pancreatitis. The dense acoustic shadowing (AS) caused by the stone load has obscured the structures of the porta hepatis lying posteriorly.

mation or oedema recognised with loss of the distinct echo-layers between mucosa and submucosa which are recognisable in the normal viscus (see Fig. 2.5).

Contact ultrasound is also useful for characterisation of lesions in patients in whom intrinsic gallbladder pathology is suspected or discovered incidentally. Cholesterolosis may thus be distinguished from adenomatous polyps, which do not typically cast acoustic shadows (Fig. 2.22). Laparoscopic ultrasound may also have a role in alerting the surgeon to the presence of unsuspected gallbladder cancer at the time of laparoscopic cholecystectomy (Fig. 2.23). In this way, an appropriate evaluation of the tumour may be

Fig. 2.20 Laparoscopic sonogram obtained with the oblique-viewing 90° sector-scanning probe placed against the undersurface of the gallbladder (GB). Compare the appearances of hypoechoic bile within the GB lumen, the sediment of echogenic sludge (S) on the posterior wall and the hyperechoic 3–4 mm diameter gallstone (GS) casting a posterior acoustic shadow.

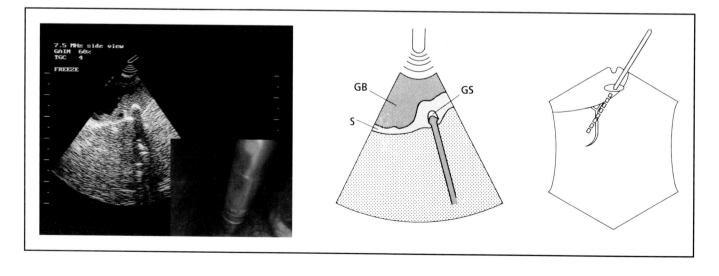

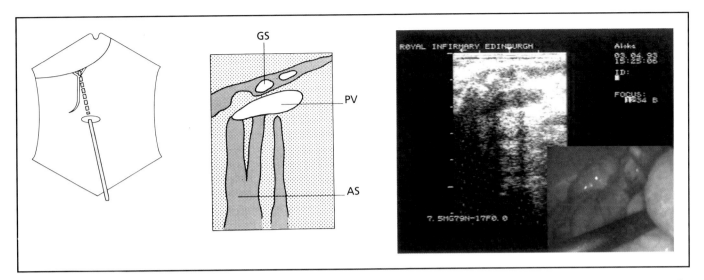

Fig. 2.21 Laparoscopic sonogram obtained with a linear-array probe placed upon the hepatoduodenal ligament. Several calculi are demonstrated within the common bile duct (GS). AS, acoustic shadows; PV, portal vein.

undertaken prior to unwitting surgical intervention which has been implicated in dissemination of the tumour [13].

Hepaticholithiasis

Whilst there remains some debate regarding the precise role of intraoperative ultrasound in the detection of stones in the extrahepatic biliary tree, there are a number of advantages in using it to exclude their presence within the intrahepatic ducts. The upper reaches of the biliary tree may not be well demonstrated by operative cholangiography if insufficient contrast is instilled.

Intraoperative ultrasonography should detect even the smallest of intrahepatic calculi since these appear highly echogenic with respect to the hepatic parenchyma (see Fig. 2.7). The associated segmental duct will invariably be dilated. It is important to note that air within the biliary tree may also produce intensely hyperechoic signals which should not be confused with intrahepatic calculi. Unfortunately, the two may coexist if there have been previous manipulations on the biliary tree. A common source of

Fig. 2.22 Laparoscopic sonogram demonstrating adenomatous polyps within a thin-walled gallbladder (GB) prior to laparoscopic cholecystectomy. Note the right kidney (RK) lying below the gallbladder, in contact with hepatic segment VI. PRPV, posterior sectoral branch of the right portal vein.

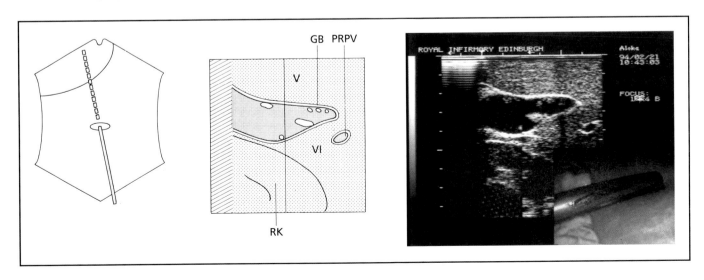

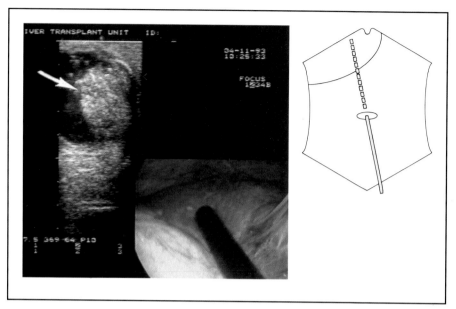

Fig. 2.23 Laparoscopic sonogram demonstrating a hyperechoic tumour mass (arrowed) extending from the gallbladder bed into the lumen in a patient with locally invasive gallbladder carcinoma.

error for the uninitiated is to mistake the obliterated umbilical vein for a calculus at the base of the falciform ligament.

Choledocholithiasis

The appearance of common duct stones is identical to that of gallbladder calculi (see Fig. 2.21). Large duct calculi are usually obvious, but the presence of duct dilatation should alert the ultrasonographer that small stones less than or equal to 5 mm in diameter may be present within the biliary tree. However, it must be recognised that duct dilatation may occur in the absence of an obstructing calculus, whilst a non-dilated duct does not necessarily exclude choledocholithiasis. Whilst duct stones are more easily detected in the supraduodenal portion of the common duct, difficulty can be encountered in defining small stones impacted in the distal common duct, especially when they are of a soft consistency and do not cast posterior acoustic shadows, or when duodenal gas interferes with the image.

Tumours in the pancreas or involving the lower bile duct are discussed in Chapter 3.

At open cholecystectomy, operative ultrasonography had been shown to be as reliable as operative cholangiography in the detection of common bile stones [6,14,15]. Sensitivity rates of between 89 and 94% and specificity rates of 98% in the detection of ductal stones by ultrasound did not convince surgeons of the need to move from routine cholangiography to intraoperative evaluation of the biliary tree. Others have suggested that the sensitivity and specificity rates of 86 and 93% for cholangiography fall short of those expected for fluoroscopic cholangiography.

Table 2.1 Comparison of operative cholangiography and laparoscopic ultrasonography (using a 7.5 MHz linear-array probe) during laparoscopic cholecystectomy in the detection of choledocholithiasis

	Operative cholangiography (*n* = 48 (54))	Laparoscopic ultrasound (*n* = 54)
True positive	5	5
True negative	40(45)	45
False positive	2	2
False negative	1(2)	2
Sensitivity	83%	71%
Specificity	95%	96%
Positive predictive value	71%	71%
Negative predictive value	98%	96%
Accuracy	94% (93%)	93%

The figures in parentheses indicate the effect on accuracy of counting the six non-successful operative cholangiograms as negative investigations.

The advent of laparoscopic cholecystectomy has resulted in a move away from routine cholangiography, heralding the use of contact ultrasound as a screening tool for the detection of common bile duct stones, of for better selecting of patients for cholangiography based upon indirect findings such as duct diameter or gallbladder stone size. Our preliminary experience using a 7.5 MHz linear-array probe [16] suggests that laparoscopic ultrasonography is at least comparable to that of routine cholangiography in the detection of common bile duct stones (Table 2.1). Of 54 patients submitted to laparoscopic ultrasonography at the time of cholecystectomy, seven patients were ultimately shown to have common bile duct stones. Cholangiograms could not be obtained in six patients, one of whom had common duct stones identified by laparoscopic ultrasonography. Overall, laparoscopic ultrasonography detected five of the seven stones with two false-positive examinations. In this early experience, the specificity of 96% was similar to reports for intraoperative ultrasonography at open cholecystectomy [14], although the lower sensitivity probably reflects an early lack of experience with the technique.

Prospective evaluation of a 90° mechanical sector-scanning laparoscopic ultrasound probe (see Fig. 2.15) has produced similar results [8]. In 60 patients so evaluated, common duct stones were detected in nine patients (one false positive and one false negative). There is little doubt that laparoscopic ultrasonography is operator dependent, and this was reflected in a 'learning curve' which was documented during the initial evaluation of this equipment. The ability of the laparoscopic ultrasonographer to satisfactorily demonstrate defined anatomical landmarks in three consecutive groups of 20 examinations is shown in Table 2.2. Larger diameter structures were easily defined at an early stage in our own experience, but the more distal structures were often difficult to locate. None the less, the early prototype lapa-roscopic ultrasound probes subsequently underwent appreciable technical refinements, and increasing experience with the sector-scanning probe

	I (n = 20)	II (n = 20)	III (n = 20)
Gallbladder	20	20	20
Suprapancreatic common duct	17	16	20
Portal vein	20	20	20
Hepatic artery	9	12	20
Intrapancreatic common duct	7	10	16
Pancreatic duct	6	5	17

Table 2.2 The learning curve — laparoscopic ultrasound identification of anatomical structures in three consecutive groups of patients undergoing cholecystectomy by one surgeon

has since enabled reliable identification of the various anatomical landmarks.

Other workers have undertaken similar work with a variety of laparoscopic ultrasound systems utilising different transducers [8,10,16–23], and the equipment specifications and corresponding results are summarised in Table 2.3. It remains to be seen which type of laparoscopic ultrasound system proves to be best suited for routine screening of the biliary tree during laparoscopic cholecystectomy, and the results of larger studies comparing laparoscopic ultrasound with operative cholangiography are awaited.

Cholangiocarcinoma

In patients submitted to laparotomy for consideration of resection of a bile duct tumour, intraoperative ultrasonography offers the opportunity to assess carefully the invasiveness of the tumour without the need to undertake a trial dissection of the structures at the porta hepatis. In such cases, the level of the obstruction in the biliary tree can be assessed and the involvement of the primary and secondary biliary confluences determined (Fig. 2.24).

Intraoperative ultrasonography may be of value in excluding the presence of hepatic metastases that have gone undetected on preoperative investigation. The clinician may have difficulty in defining the lesion when diffuse and sclerotic, and when found to be isoechoic with the liver parenchyma. However, solid tumours may be more easily recognised by the presence of a hyperechoic mass lesion, and invasion of the liver, and the caudate lobe in particular, may be delineated. Vascular involvement or displacement is frequent with such tumours and careful assessment should be undertaken with the ultrasound probe positioned in several planes. In this way, the relationship of the tumour with the hepatic arterial and portal vein branches can be assessed.

There is a strong rationale for performing preoperative laparoscopic staging with laparoscopic ultrasound in the evaluation of patients with proximal bile duct obstruction. There is no doubting the value of laparoscopy in the detection of peritoneal and overt hepatic metastases from such tumours, but adequate evaluation of lesions involving the confluence of the hepatic ducts has, until now, not been possible. The laparoscopic ultrasound examination can also yield information concerning local invasion and regional

Table 2.3 Laparoscopic ultrasound examination of the common bile duct (CBD) during laparoscopic cholecystectomy. (Courtesy of [24], with permission)

Reference	LapUS probe specifications	Number of cases	Lap US-detected CBD stones	Comment
Ascher *et al.* [17]	12.5 MHz 360° sectoral (Diasonics)	20	None	CBD stones successfully detected in a pig model
Goletti *et al.* [18]	7.5 MHz linear array (Aloka UST–5521–7.5)	20	4	Forward- and side-viewing probes
	7.5 MHz 90° sectoral (Endomedix LaparoScan)	10		
Greig *et al.* [16]	7.5 MHz linear array (Aloka UST–5521–7.5)	54	5 2 False negatives 2 False positives	
Jakimowicz [10]	7.5 MHz linear array (Aloka UST–5522–7.5)	145	12 1 False negative	Doppler/ colour flow facility
John *et al.* [8]	7.5 MHz 90° sectoral (Endomedix LaparoScan)	60	9 1 False negative 1 False positive	Forward- and side-viewing probes
Machi *et al.* [19]	7.5 MHz linear array (Aloka UST–5522–7.5)	25	1	Doppler/ colour flow facility
Röthlin *et al.* [20,21]	5.5 MHz 360° sectoral (Brüel & Kjoer)	100	4 2 False positives	Bile duct anomaly 22% Arterial anomaly 20%
Stiegmann *et al.* [22]	7.5 MHz linear array (Tetrad Inc.)	31	5	
Yamamoto *et al.* [23]	7.5 MHz linear array (Tetrad Inc.)	5	None	Doppler/ colour flow facility
Yamashita *et al.* [11]	7.5 MHz flexible convex array (Aloka)	45	1	Doppler/ colour flow facility

nodal spread of the tumour, thereby enabling the surgeon to determine the appropriate management policy at an early stage (Fig. 2.25).

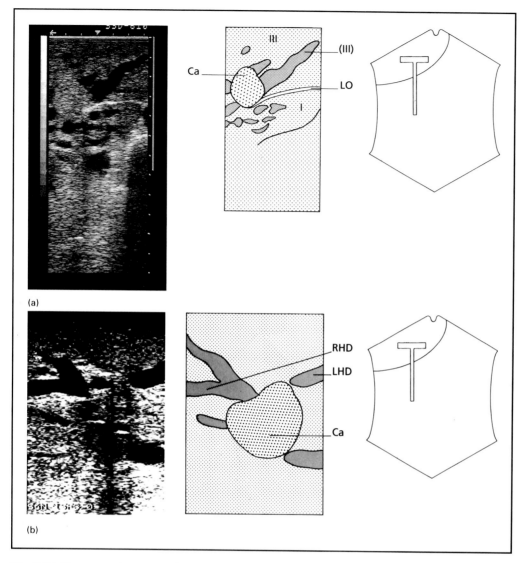

Fig. 2.24 Transverse intraoperative sonograms obtained during laparotomy and operative assessment of resectability in patients with hilar cholangiocarcinoma. (a) A 20-mm-diameter cholangiocarcinoma (Ca) occluding the segment III and I duct systems is shown. It was possible to perform a left hepatectomy with curative intent. (b) A 40-mm tumour mass was identified infiltrating the hilar plate and liver with right portal vein occlusion. Note separation of the distended right (RHD) and left (LHD) duct systems, although the secondary biliary confluences were patent (Bismuth type II stricture). A palliative segment III cholangiojejunostomy was performed having localised a distended segment III biliary radicle. LO, lesser omentum.

Benign biliary stricture

It can often be difficult to determine the precise aetiology of the obstruction of the biliary tree before surgical intervention. In such cases, operative ultrasonography may be of value in characterising the nature and site of the obstruction. Laparoscopy and laparoscopic ultrasonography have been used

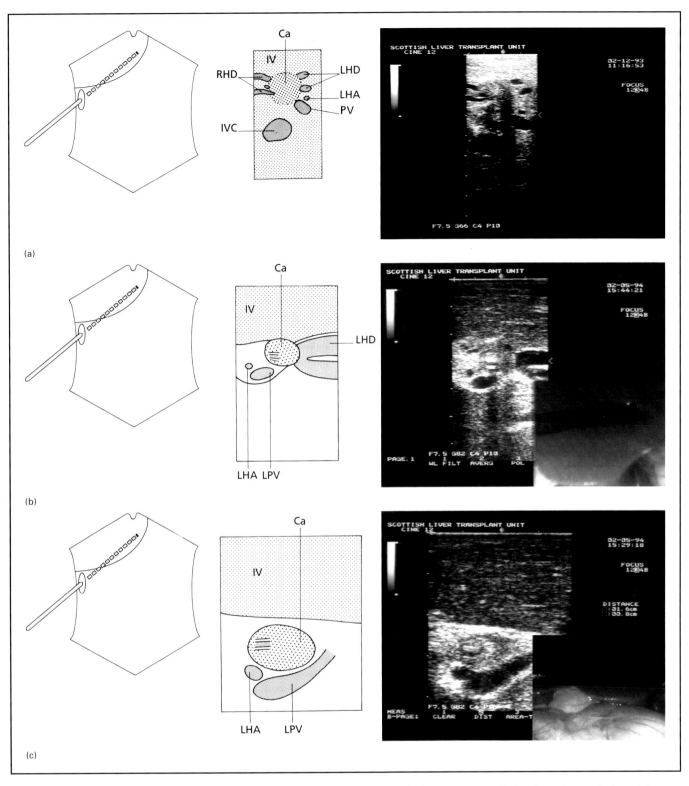

Fig. 2.25 Laparoscopic ultrasound evaluation of hilar cholangiocarcinoma. The linear-array probe has been inserted via a right flank port to provide transversely orientated sonograms through hepatic segment IV. (a) A small but irresectable tumour mass (Ca) invading the hilar plate and extending bilaterally to occlude the secondary biliary confluences has been defined. (b) A 15-mm-diameter hyperechoic cholangiocarcinoma is demonstrated extending to the secondary biliary confluence of the left duct system (LHD). There was no evidence of invasion of the liver, or adjacent hepatic artery or portal vein (PV) branches. The patient later underwent left hepatectomy with curative intent. Note the highly echogenic biliary stent traversing the tumour mass. (c) Same examination as (b), but with the probe slightly rotated to demonstrate the patency of the left portal vein (LPV) and hepatic artery (LHA). IVC, inferior vena cava; RHD, right hepatic duct.

in patients in whom there is doubt as to whether the diagnosis in the jaundiced patient is one of cholangiocarcinoma or primary sclerosing cholangitis. The ultrasonographic appearances of the two conditions may not differ greatly, but vascular invasion can be assessed and an attempt made at targeted biopsy.

Although laparoscopic ultrasonography has little role, if any, in the management of bile duct injury, the hepatobiliary surgeon may find it useful to have an operative ultrasound probe available to evaluate the injury or subsequent stricture at the time of intended repair (Fig. 2.8). The linear-array ultrasound probe will confirm the precise level of obstruction. Although preoperative cholangiography may assist in determining the severity of the injury, evaluation of the biliary tree at the time of surgical intervention is useful in demonstrating whether there is any extrahepatic duct dilatation proximal to the stricture, and in planning the operative strategy for reconstruction of the biliary tree.

References

1 Knight PR, Newell JA. Operative use of ultrasonics in cholelithiasis. *Lancet* 1963; i: 1023–5.

2 Eiseman B, Greenlaw RH, Gallagher JQ. Localization of common bile duct stones by ultrasound. *Arch Surg* 1965; 91: 195–9.

3 Lane RJ, Glazer G. Intra-operative B-mode ultrasound scanning of the extra-hepatic biliary system and pancreas. *Lancet* 1980; 2: 334–7.

4 Sigel B, Coelho JCU, Spigos DG, *et al.* Real-time ultrasonography during biliary surgery. *Radiology* 1980; 137: 531–3.

5 Sigel B, Coelho JCU, Nyhus LM, *et al.* Detection of pancreatic tumours by ultrasound during surgery. *Arch Surg* 1982; 117: 1058–61.

6 Jakimowicz JJ, Rutten H, Jürgens PJ, Carol EJ. Comparison of operative ultrasonography and radiography in screening of the common bile duct for calculi. *World J Surg* 1987; 11: 628–34.

7 Mosnier H, Audy J-CR, Boche O, Guivarc'h M. Intraoperative sonography during cholecystectomy for gallstones. *Surg Gynecol Obstet* 1992; 174: 469–73.

8 John TG, Banting SW, Pye S, Paterson-Brown S, Garden OJ. Preliminary experience with intracorporeal laparoscopic ultrasonography using a sector scanning probe: a prospective comparison with intraoperative cholangiography in the detection of choledocholithiasis. *Surg Endosc* 1994; 8: 1176–81.

9 Berci G, Sackier JM, Paz-Partlow M. Routine or selected intraoperative cholangiography during laparoscopic cholecystectomy. *Am J Surg* 1991; 161: 355–60.

10 Jakimowicz JJ. Intraoperative ultrasonography during minimal access surgery. *J Roy Col Surg Edin* 1993; 38: 231–8.

11 Yamashita Y, Kurohiji T, Hayashi J, Kimitsuki H, Hiraki M, Kakegawa T. Intraoperative ultrasonography during laparoscopic cholecystectomy. *Surg Laparosc Endosc* 1993; 3: 167–71.

12 Röthlin M, Largiadèr F. New, mobile-tip ultrasound probe for laparoscopic sonography. *Surg Endosc* 1994; 8: 805–8.

13 Fong Y, Brennan M, Turnbull A, Colt DG, Blumgart LH. Gallbladder cancer discovered during laparoscopic surgery. Potential for iatrogenic tumor dissemination. *Arch Surg* 1993; 128: 1054–6.

14 Sigel B, Machi J, Beitler JC, *et al.* Comparative accuracy of operative ultrasonography in detecting common duct calculi. *Surgery* 1983; 94: 715–20.

15 Sigel B, Coelho JCU, Nyhus LM, Donahue PE, Velasco JM, Spigos DG. Comparison of cholangiography and ultrasonography in the operative screening of the common bile duct. *World J Surg* 1982; 6: 440–4.

16 Greig JD, John TG, Mahadaven M, Garden OJ. Laparoscopic ultrasonography in the evaluation of the biliary tree during laparoscopic cholecystectomy. *Br J Surg* 1994; 81: 1202–6.

17 Ascher SM, Evans SRT, Goldberg JA, *et al.* Intraoperative bile duct sonography during laparoscopic cholecystectomy: experience with a 12.5-MHz catheter-based US probe. *Radiology* 1992; 185: 493–6.

18 Goletti O, Buccianti P, Decanini L, *et al.* Intraoperative sonography of biliary tree during laparoscopic cholecystectomy. *Surg Laparosc Endosc* 1994; 4: 9–12.

19 Machi J, Sigel B, Zaren HA, *et al.* Technique of ultrasound examination during laparoscopic cholecystectomy. *Surg Endosc* 1993; 7: 544–9.

20 Röthlin MA, Schlumpf R, Largiadèr F. Laparoscopic sonography. An alternative to routine intraoperative cholangiography? *Arch Surg* 1994; 129: 694–700.

21 Röthlin M, Largiadèr F. The anatomy of the hepatoduodenal ligament in laparoscopic sonography. *Surg Endosc* 1994; 8: 173–80.

22 Stiegmann RV, McIntyre RC, Pearlman NW. Laparoscopic intracorporeal ultrasound. An alternative to cholangiography? *Surg Endosc* 1994; 8: 167–72.

23 Yamamoto M, Stiegmann GV, Durham J, *et al.* Laparoscopy-guided intracorporeal ultrasound accurately delineates hepatobiliary anatomy. *Surg Endosc* 1993; 7: 325–30.

24 John TG, Garden OJ. Ultrasonography in laparoscopy. In: Brooks D, ed. *Current Review of Laparoscopy*, 2nd edn. Philadelphia: Current Medicine, 1995 (in press).

3: Intraoperative and Laparoscopic Ultrasound of the Liver

In spite of the many improvements in preoperative radiological investigations which are aimed at ensuring that malignancy is confined to the liver, suspected hepatic lesions may not be defined with sufficient accuracy [1]. For most surgeons the intention is to identify individuals with tumour that can be resected without risk to the patient and with the best prospects of cure. None the less, it is not uncommon to find that a resection which has been undertaken with curative intent, turns out to have been palliative at best [2,3]. Hepatobiliary surgeons in Europe have long been aware of the potential advantages of employing ultrasound in the operating room. In patients submitted to laparotomy, operative ultrasonography can provide accurate information on the degree of hepatic involvement by a tumour and can facilitate hepatic resection [4]. Furthermore, operative ultrasonography has resulted in therapeutic advances as it provides a means of visualising and gaining access to the intrahepatic portal venous system [5,6].

In the same way that hepatobiliary surgeons have embraced ultrasound technology in the treatment of hepatic malignancy, so general surgeons have looked towards this technique in the detection of hepatic involvement from other intra-abdominal neoplasms. It has long been recognised, for example, that the single most important determinant of survival of patients undergoing apparently curative resection of colorectal tumours is the presence of hepatic involvement [7,8]. Such infiltration of the liver may go undetected by preoperative scanning and, indeed, deep intrahepatic lesions may easily be missed by the surgeon's palpating hand at laparotomy [9]. Detection of these 'occult' metastases is an important part of the overall management of the patient and has been greatly facilitated by the use of intraoperative ultrasonography [1].

With the arrival of minimal access surgery it was inevitable that the relative advantages of diagnostic laparoscopy and intraoperative ultrasonography be combined in an attempt to improve the assessment of intra-abdominal malignancy [10–12]. The value of laparoscopy in the detection of small peritoneal and liver metastases has been well documented [11,13–17]. Some have recognised that the laparoscopic demonstration of extrahepatic and bilobar spread of disease in patients under consideration for resection of hepatocellular carcinoma can also avoid unnecessary operative intervention [18,19]. None the less, laparoscopy is limited as a staging tool inasmuch as the detailed view of the abdominal viscera obtained by the laparoscopist is restricted to visible organ surfaces. The development of high-resolution ultrasound transducers which can be placed in direct apposition with the liver capsule through standard laparoscopic ports permits detailed examination and promises to revolutionise the assessment of intra-abdominal malignancy [11,20].

This chapter will provide detailed descriptions of the technique of intraoperative and laparoscopic ultrasonography, highlighting their role in the assessment of hepatic lesions. In order to emphasise the potential of the newer technology of laparoscopic ultrasound, the use of operative ultrasound will be discussed first.

Anatomy (Figs 3.1 and 3.2)

Couinaud's classical description of the liver anatomy is ideally suited for ultrasound examination of the liver (Fig. 3.1) [21,22]. The intrahepatic vascular structures are readily identified by ultrasound (Fig. 3.2) and any associated pathology can be accurately localised.

The vena cava lies to the right of the midline behind the liver and may be partially surrounded by the hepatic parenchyma. It is compressible and its diameter will vary according to the respiratory cycle. The confluence of the hepatic veins with the vena cava can be identified at the superior aspect of the liver. Since the hepatic veins lie outwith Glisson's capsule, they appear as hypoechoic areas with only an ill-defined wall. Blood flow may be observed within the lumen as the cardiac pulsations are transmitted to the veins. In almost all cases, the left and middle hepatic veins join the vena cava as a common trunk (see Fig. 3.1). The left hepatic vein is formed from a number of smaller tributaries with the main vessel running between segments II and III within the left lobe (see Fig. 3.2).

The middle hepatic vein runs along a plane (principal portal fissure) which separates the two hemilivers with their respective portal venous and hepatic

Fig. 3.1 Couinaud's segmental anatomy of the liver: (a) anterior and (b) right lateral views. RHV, right hepatic vein; MHV, middle hepatic vein; LHV, left hepatic vein; IVC, interior vena cava.

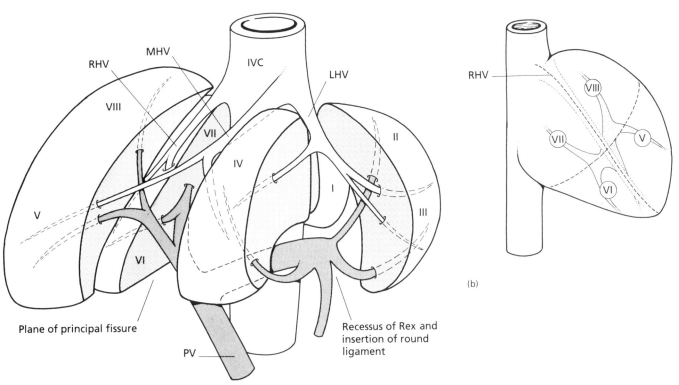

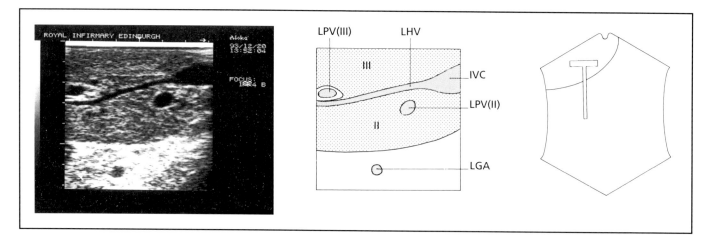

arterial blood supply. The middle hepatic vein is formed from two substantial veins which arise anteriorly in segments IV and V. In almost half of the cases there is a further substantial vein which drains the superior portion of segment IV and joins the main middle hepatic vein at a variable distance from the vena cava. On occasion, a small accessory vein will drain direct from either segment IV or VIII into the vena cava.

The right hepatic vein enters the vena cava at its right border and slightly inferior to the other two veins. This vein lies between the anterior (segments V and VIII) and posterior (segments VI and VII) sectors of the right hemiliver (see Fig. 3.1). In less than 20% of cases there is an accessory vein which drains segment VI and enters the vena cava at the level of the hilus. This anatomical variant to the venous drainage of the liver may be useful in undertaking anatomical resections aimed at preserving segment VI and yet involving sacrifice of the main right hepatic vein [23,24].

There are a variable number of small hepatic veins draining directly from the caudate lobe (segment I) to the vena cava and which are not often visible on ultrasound scanning.

The portal pedicle is enveloped in a fibrous sheath which is derived from Glisson's capsule. The capsule thickens considerably at the hilus to become the hilar plate (Fig. 3.3). The vessels therefore differ from the hepatic veins on ultrasound scanning as a result of their hyperechoic wall. The portal vein branches are accompanied by branches of the hepatic artery and by the biliary radicles. The bile ducts are anterior and superior to the portal vein branches and the arteries pass between the two, although their small size and tortuous course often makes it difficult for them to be identified on scanning.

The left portal pedicle pursues an extrahepatic course giving branches posteriorly to the caudate lobe (segment I) and to segment II. It passes anteriorly to end at the round ligament as the recess of Rex. At this level it divides into the terminal segment III and IV branches.

The right portal pedicle leaves the hilus to the right and follows a short extrahepatic course before dividing into two sectoral trunks, the anterior of which supplies segments V and VIII between the middle and right hepatic veins. The remaining trunk passes posteriorly before dividing into branches to segments VI and VII which are situated posterior to the right hepatic vein.

Fig. 3.2 Intraoperative sonogram obtained with a 5 MHz linear-array T-probe placed in a transverse/oblique orientation upon the left hepatic lobe. The left hepatic vein (LHV) is demonstrated draining into the inferior vena cava (IVC) posteriorly, and separates segments II and III. The portal venous branches to segments II and III from the left portal vein are shown in cross-section (LPV(II) and LPV(III)). Note the sinusoidal character of the hepatic vein, whereas the portal venous branches are invested with a hyperechoic fascial sheath. LGA, left gastric artery.

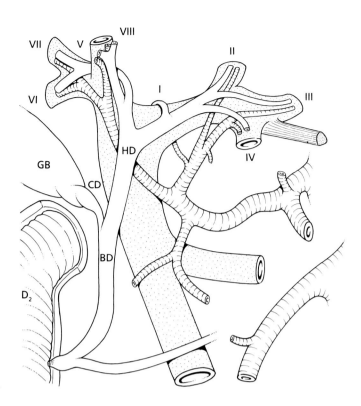

Fig. 3.3 The sectoral and segmental branches of the hilus. The accompanying branches of the hepatic artery and portal vein are shown. BD, common bile duct; CD, cystic duct; D₂, second part of duodenum; GB, gallbladder; HD, common hepatic duct.

Ultrasound examination of the normal liver

The liver can be evaluated with either a linear-array or sectoral probe. The advantage of the latter type of probe is that the small diameter probe tip requires only to be in contact with a limited part of the liver surface. The main disadvantage is the loss of definition in the far field with loss of two-point discrimination. It is generally easier for the surgeon at open operation to employ a linear-array ultrasound probe which can be placed flat on the liver. The surgeon can readily identify the intrahepatic structures and establish their relationship with each other. It is our own practice to use a T-shaped 5 MHz linear-array probe at open surgery and the evaluation of the liver using this instrument will be described. A 5 MHz transducer will provide less resolution but better penetration of the liver, although we have favoured the use of a 7.5 MHz linear-array transducer at laparoscopy.

Intraoperative ultrasonography

The examination of the liver commences with the probe placed transversely over the anterior portion of the quadrate lobe (segment IV). The vena cava will be identified at the back of the liver. With the probe inclined superiorly the hepatic veins can be readily recognised as they converge posteriorly to enter the vena cava (Fig. 3.4). The veins are characterised by their position and almost indistinct hyperechoic wall. The probe can be gradually moved over the quadrate lobe (segment IV) to improve the visualisation of each individual vein and to identify any venous anomaly (Fig. 3.5). The probe can be rotated and placed sagittally to determine the relationship of the vein with the individual segmental branches of the portal pedicle and any associated lesions (Fig. 3.6).

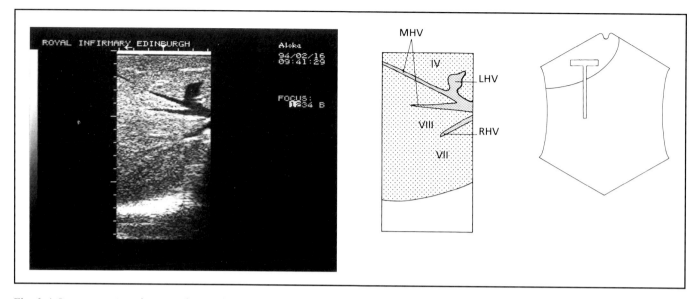

Fig. 3.4 Intraoperative ultrasound scan through the quadrate lobe (IV) demonstrating the confluence of the left (LHV) and middle (MHV) hepatic veins at the inferior vena cava (IVC). The right hepatic vein (RHV) is also seen and enters the IVC separately. The adjacent hepatic segments are numbered.

The portal vein and its division into right and left branches can be examined by maintaining the position of the probe on the inferior portion of the quadrate lobe (segment IV). The right hemiliver can be examined by following the right branch of the portal vein peripherally by gradual movement of the probe over the liver, combined with gentle changes in the angle of the probe. The anterior sectoral branch and its segmental divisions can be located between the right and middle hepatic veins. Similarly, the posterior sectoral branch and its segmental divisions will be located behind the right hepatic vein (Fig. 3.7).

Fig. 3.5 Transverse intraoperative sonogram through the quadrate lobe of the liver. An accessory right hepatic vein (ARHV) is seen joining the inferior vena cava (IVC) below the insertion of the right hepatic vein and at the level of the portal venous bifurcation. The right portal vein (RPV), its posterior sectoral (PSPV) branch and the left portal vein (LPV) are also shown. Ao, aorta; LGA, left gastric artery; VC, vertebral column. Probe position is the same as that used in Fig. 3.4.

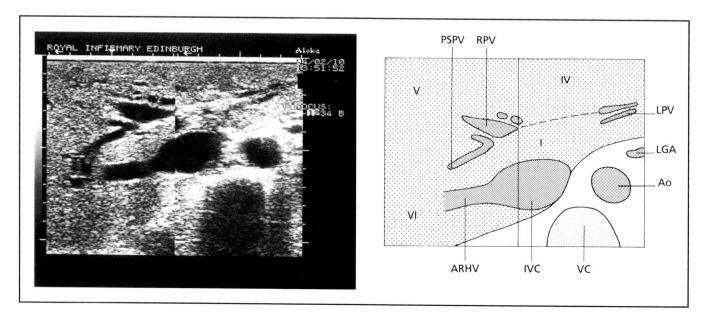

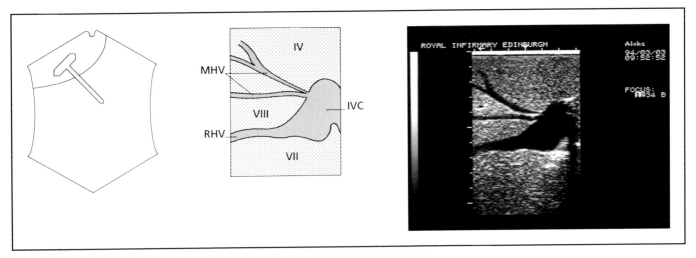

Fig. 3.6 An oblique view taken with the transducer placed transversely on the quadrate lobe (IV) demonstrating a bifid middle hepatic vein (MHV) entering the inferior vena cava (IVC) separately from the right hepatic vein (RHV). The MHV separates the posterior segments of the right hemiliver (VII and VIII) from the quadrate lobe (IV).

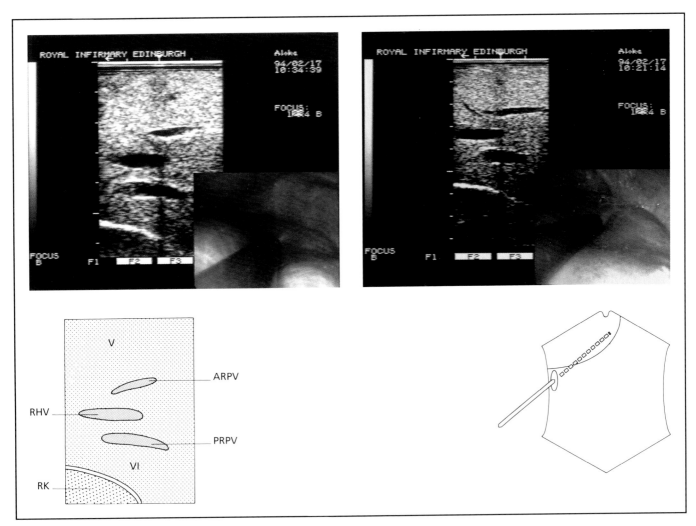

Fig. 3.7 Laparoscopic sonogram obtained with the 7.5 MHz linear-array probe placed obliquely over the right hemiliver. The right hepatic vein (RHV) separates the anterior (V) and posterior (VI) sectors of the right liver, supplied respectively by the anterior (ARPV) and posterior (PRPV) sectoral branches of the right portal vein. The right kidney (RK) lies posterior to segment VI.

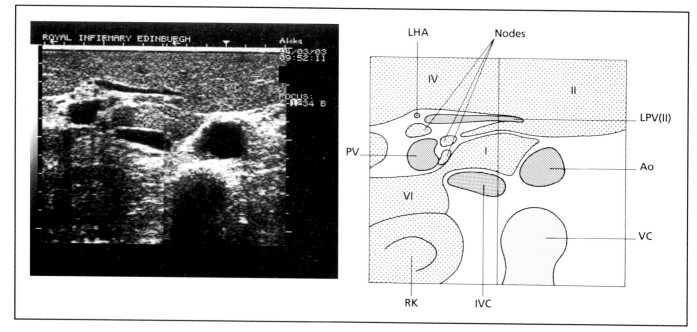

Fig. 3.8 Transverse sonogram through the quadrate lobe of the liver. The left branch of the portal vein (LPV) courses anterior to the caudate lobe (I), which separates it from the inferior vena cava (IVC), aorta (Ao) and vertebral column (VC), and terminates as the segment II radicle. The right kidney (RK) lies immediately posterior to segment VI. Lymphadenopathy surrounding the portal vein (PV) has also been demonstrated. LHA, left hepatic artery. Probe position is the same as that used in Fig. 3.9.

As these structures are identified the right kidney will be observed posteriorly. It is useful to compare the echoity of the two organs since this is similar when the liver is not diseased. As the probe is passed inferiorly over segments IV and V, the gallbladder will come into view as a hypoechoic structure with a densely hyperechoic wall. Its longitudinal axis will lie in the same principal plane as the middle hepatic vein.

The main branches of the left portal pedicle can be well seen with the probe placed on the lateral aspect of segment IV (Fig. 3.8). However, a complete examination of the left lobe will require the transducer to be transferred to the other side of the falciform ligament on to segment III, so that the left hepatic vein can be traced as it runs between segments II and III. The left portal pedicle can be followed as it passes to the left and anteriorly to reach the obliterated umbilical vein passing within the round ligament. The branches to segments I and II can be seen passing directly into the hepatic parenchyma. The lesser omentum appears as a hyperechoic line separating the caudate lobe (segment I) and segment II (Fig. 3.9). The principal supplying vessels to segments IV and III can be seen to pass to the left and right, and other smaller segmental branches can be located more posteriorly.

The structures at the porta hepatis can be evaluated by tracing the portal vein back from its bifurcation to its origin at the confluence of the superior mesenteric and splenic veins. By placing the ultrasound probe on segment IV, all of these structures should be visualised without the need to apply the probe directly on to the porta hepatis. It may be necessary to instill some saline or interpose a saline filled pouch between the probe and the portal structures to avoid loss of detail immediately beneath the probe ('near field') if the liver is not used as a stand-off ('acoustic window') (Fig. 3.10).

In the majority of cases it is possible to identify the common hepatic duct as it lies anterolateral to the portal vein with the proper hepatic artery on its

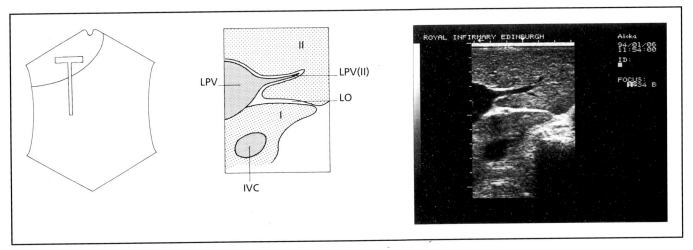

Fig. 3.9 Transverse intraoperative sonogram showing the termination of the left portal vein (LPV) in the recessus of Rex, along with the insertion of the lesser omentum (LO), which separates segments I and II. IVC, inferior vena cava; LPV(II), left portal venous radicle to segment II.

medial aspect (Fig. 3.11). The right and left hepatic ducts can be seen as they emerge from the liver substance, although it is often difficult to define the non-dilated duct within the liver substance. The arterial anatomy can be variable and the bifurcation of the proper hepatic artery may occur at almost any level. Similarly, the relationship of the right hepatic artery to the bile duct is inconsistent. It may pass behind or in front of the hepatic duct, and in those cases where the hepatic artery arises from the superior mesenteric artery, the right hepatic artery will invariably course posterolateral to the ductal structures. It may also be possible to recognise lymph nodes at the porta hepatis.

Laparoscopic ultrasonography

The examination technique for both linear-array and mechanical sectoral probes will be described since there are certain differences between the two.

Linear array

The technique of laparoscopic ultrasonography of the liver is based on that of intraoperative ultrasonography, although the linear-array probe enters the peritoneal cavity in a longitudinal direction as opposed to the transverse orientation previously described for open surgery. Access to the peritoneal cavity is gained through two 10/11 mm ports which are placed at the umbilicus and to the right of this port in the midclavicular or anterior axillary line. It is preferable to use disposable ports to enable safe passage of the ultrasound probe, the surface of which may be inadvertently damaged by the metal spring-valves of traditional non-disposable ports. The laparoscope and laparoscopic ultrasound probe can be interchanged between the two ports to provide different views of the liver and to accomodate the varying placement of the probe on the liver surface.

Following the insertion of the laparoscope through the umbilical port, displacement of the liver or the structures at the porta hepatis is best avoided

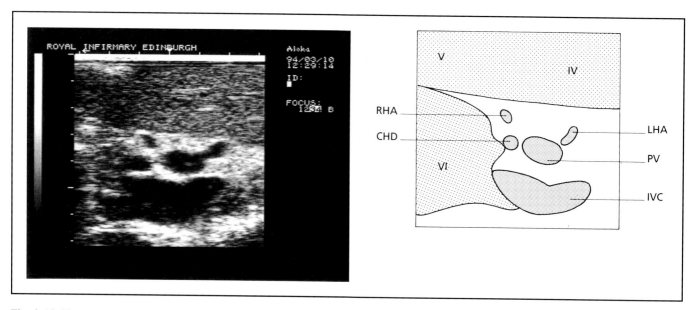

Fig. 3.10 Transverse intraoperative sonogram through the anterior segments of the right liver (IV and V), demonstrating the hilar structures. The portal vein (PV) lies anterior to the inferior vena cava (IVC); the common hepatic duct (CHD) lies laterally in the free edge of the hepatoduodenal ligament; and the common hepatic artery has divided into its branches to the right and left hemiliver, respectively (RHA and LHA). Probe position is the same as that used in Fig. 3.11.

to prevent insufflation of carbon dioxide gas in the subhepatic space. The presence of gas in the tissue spaces may interfere with subsequent imaging of the structures at the porta hepatis. Instillation of fluid may overcome this problem and can be sampled by aspiration for cytological analysis.

The laparoscope is transferred from the umbilical to the right lateral port and the ultrasound probe is passed through the umbilical cannula, avoiding inadvertent damage to the transducer by the port's flap valve (Fig. 3.12). The 7.5 MHz laparoscopic ultrasound probe is placed under direct laparoscopic visualisation on the diaphragmatic surface of segment IV (quadrate lobe). This will enable the surgeon to visualise the portal vein and its bifur-

Fig. 3.11 Transverse intraoperative sonogram through the quadrate lobe of the liver, demonstrating the main portal vein (PV), common hepatic artery (CHA) and common hepatic duct (CHD) in the free edge of the hepatoduodenal ligament. An aberrant branch from the right hepatic artery (RPHA) supplying the posterior sector of the right hemiliver is seen passing posterolateral to these structures. IVC, inferior vena cava; LPV, left portal vein; VC, vertebral column.

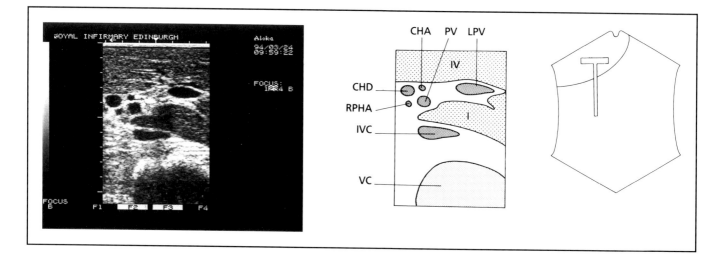

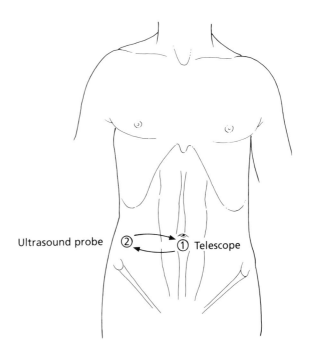

Fig. 3.12 Diagrammatic representation of the position of the ports, laparoscope and laparoscopic ultrasound probe during evaluation of the liver.

Fig. 3.13 Laparoscopic sonogram through the quadrate lobe of the liver showing the structures of hepatic pedicle in longitudinal section. The common hepatic duct (CHD) is shown lying anterolateral to the portal vein (PV) and separated from the inferior vena cava (IVC) and aorta (Ao) by the caudate lobe (Seg I). The origin of the middle hepatic vein (MHV) within segment IV is demonstrated.

cation at the outset of the examination and so allow the surgeon to explore the liver from this landmark.

As at open surgery the ultrasound probe can be displaced gradually over the right hemiliver. Rotation of the probe to the patient's right side will allow the surgeon to explore the right hemiliver itself, whilst rotation in the opposite direction should bring the structures at the porta hepatis into view. Examination of the left lobe will require the surgeon to move the probe to the other side of the falciform ligament on to segments II and III.

The portal vein is separated from the vena cava by the caudate lobe (segment I). Blood flow may be evident within both vessels and the vena cava will often transmit cardiac pulsations (Fig. 3.13). The hepatic artery and common hepatic duct lie anterior to the portal vein and the artery is recognised by its pulsation.

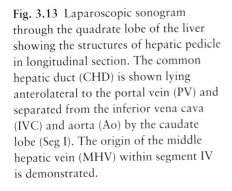

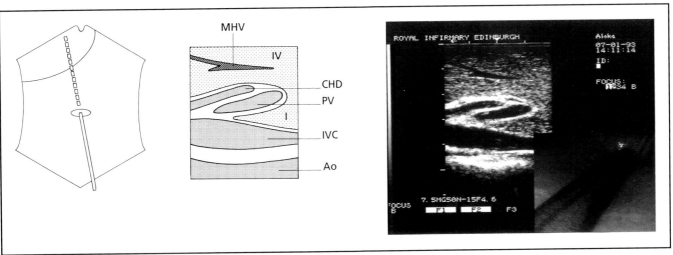

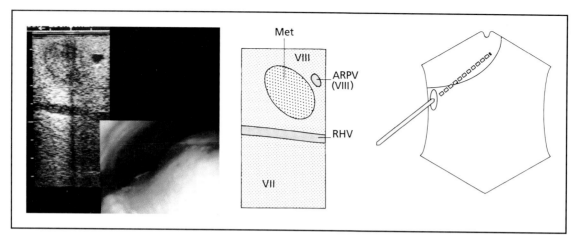

The anterior and posterior sectoral divisions of the right branch of the portal vein can be followed out into the right hemiliver although the associated ducts may not be readily visible unless these are dilated (Fig. 3.14). They and the arterial branches will lie anterior to the portal vein branches. The left branch of the portal vein and its segmental branches may be followed as they run to the left lobe of the liver.

Laparoscopic evaluation of the liver is undertaken normally with the intention of detecting lesions within the hepatic parenchyma. None the less, knowledge of the position of the vessels will ensure that these are not mistaken for an intrahepatic lesion. Identification of the middle hepatic vein is useful before examination of the right hemiliver. The ultrasound probe is advanced from the junction of segments IV and V in the region of the gallbladder towards the vena cava. The middle hepatic vein will be seen running from the inferior and anterior aspect of the liver to the upper reaches of the liver posteriorly as the vein joins the vena cava at its confluence with the left hepatic vein (Fig. 3.15). Displacement or rotation of the probe to the right and left will bring the right and left hepatic veins into view.

Further examination of the liver can be undertaken with the transducer placed beneath the liver, but the resultant scans can be a little difficult to orientate (Fig. 3.16).

Sectoral probe

It has been our practice to employ routinely linear-array probes to evaluate the liver. The currently available sectoral ultrasound probes are designed more for the assessment of shallow organs such as in the examination of the biliary tree and the pancreas. Such probes can, however, be employed in the screening of the liver for metastatic disease. Access can be achieved by a number of ways, but adequate views can be obtained by using an oblique-viewing ultrasound probe inserted through an umbilical or right lumbar port. Because of the limited penetration of such probes it may be necessary to examine the liver on both its anterior and inferior surfaces (Fig. 3.17). It is more difficult for the surgeon to orientate to the anatomy of the liver than with a linear-array probe, but the vessels can be recognised in the same way as described above.

Fig. 3.14 Oblique laparoscopic sonogram through the posterior aspect of the right hemiliver in the long axis of the right hepatic vein (RHV), which is shown separating segments VII and VIII. A hypoechoic metastasis (Met) lies adjacent to the anterior sectoral branch of the right portal vein (ARPV) which passes in the opposite plane and is seen in cross-section.

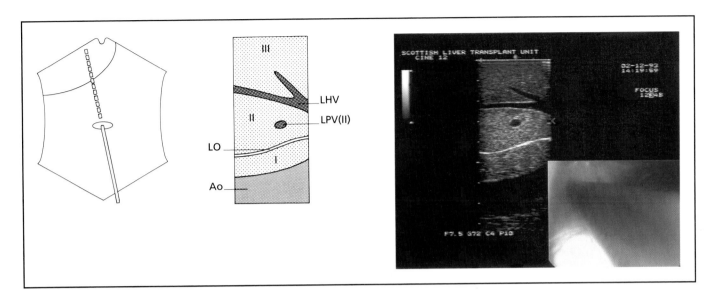

Fig. 3.15 Laparoscopic sonogram through the left hepatic lobe, demonstrating the left hepatic vein (LHV) passing posteriorly (LPV(II)) towards the vena cava. The segmental portal venous branch within segment II is separated from the caudate lobe (I) and aorta (Ao) by the hyperechoic fascial insertion of the lesser omentum (LO).

Fig. 3.16 Laparoscopic sonogram with the ultrasound probe placed beneath the left hepatic lobe and scanning upwards. The insertion of the lesser omentum appears as a hyperechoic plane separating segments I and II.

Hepatic pathology

The ability to evaluate areas of interest in the liver in real time is one of the strengths of intraoperative and laparoscopic ultrasonography. The complex acoustic shadows cast by structures in the liver can make the interpretation of static views difficult. Operative ultrasound can visualise the same area from a number of different angles enabling a more complete assessment of the lesion than can be obtained by preoperative scanning. It should, however, be borne in mind that small superficial lesions may lie in the dead zone of the scanning head and may only be detected if the probe is placed on the posterior aspect of the lobe or if a stand-off is employed.

Hepatic cysts

Intrahepatic cysts are not uncommonly found on routine scanning of the liver and are said to be present in up to 10% of the normal population [25].

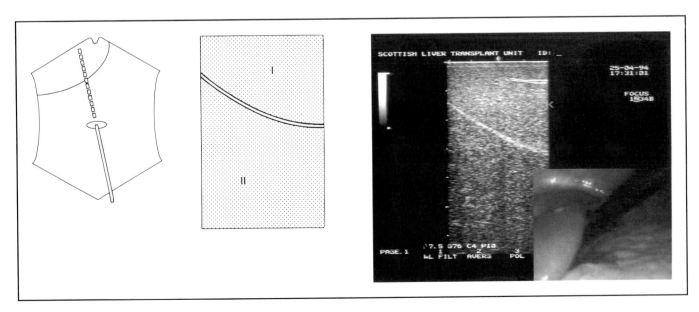

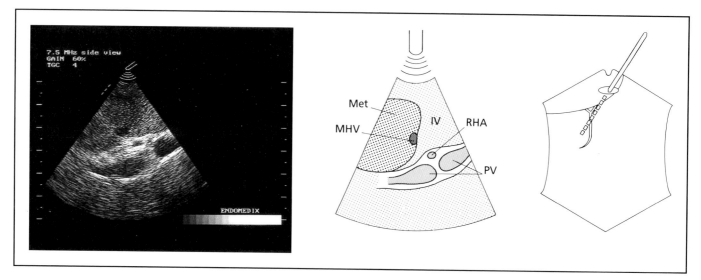

They are easily recognised on scanning by their ultrasound features alone. They may be multiple and are generally smooth and spherical. These benign cysts are uniloculate and have a thin uniform wall of low echoity. The ultrasound signal passes unimpeded through the sonolucent cyst and produces an image of relative enhancement directly behind the cyst (Fig. 3.18). On occasion the cyst fluid contains small cholesterol crystals which appear as 'snowflakes' within the cyst.

Conversely, hydatid cysts are also sonolucent but the fluid-filled cyst has a well-defined, often calcified, capsule which produces a hyperechoic image on scanning. Small cysts may be observed on scanning and are often embedded in the wall of the main cyst. These appearances can be mimicked by a benign hepatic cyst which has previously been infected or been the site of previous haemorrhage.

Operative ultrasonography is of value at open surgery when large symptomatic non-parasitic cysts require to be deroofed. The scan will assist the surgeon in planning the extent of the excision of the wall and identify adjacent vascular structures (Fig. 3.19).

Fig. 3.17 Laparoscopic sonogram of the liver using a 7.5 MHz 90° sectoral-scanning probe. A centrally situated solitary metastasis (Met) is identified astride segments IV and V anteriorly abutting the middle hepatic vein (MHV) immediately above the bifurcation of the portal vein (PV). RHA, right hepatic artery.

Fig. 3.18 The characteristic features of a benign intrahepatic cyst, which was not visible laparoscopically, are demonstrated by laparoscopic ultrasound. There is no defined wall surrounding the fluid-filled cyst which appears anechoic and is associated with posterior acoustic enhancement. PV, portal vein.

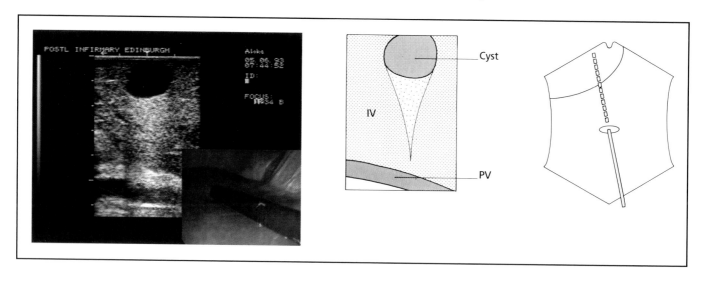

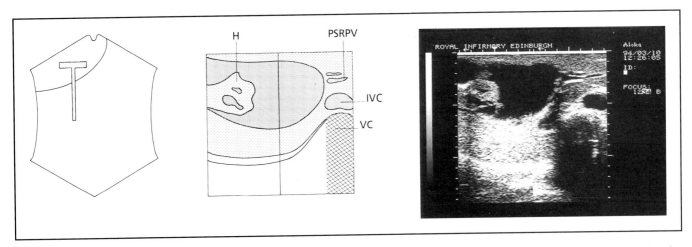

Fig. 3.19 Intraoperative sonogram demonstrating a large cyst situated in the right hemiliver approached closely by the posterior sectoral branch of the right portal vein (PSRPV). The solid component within the cyst cavity represents hyperechoic haematoma (H) following previous attempts at percutaneous aspiration. Compare the dense acoustic shadows cast by the vertebral column with the acoustic enhancement posterior to the cyst. IVC, inferior vena cava; VC, vertebral column.

Laparoscopic ultrasonography has assumed greater importance in the management of non-parasitic cysts, since it can be used to assess their relationship to the vessels during laparoscopic deroofing of such lesions (Fig. 3.20). The ultrasound examination is of particular value in locating the major vessels as more superficial cysts are cleared and the deeper cysts require to be located and drained.

Haemangioma

Arteriovenous malformations are found with increasing frequency during ultrasound scanning of the liver with high-resolution probes. In contrast to liver cysts, they appear as dense echoic areas in normal liver. There is diffuse echoity throughout the lesion which displays a minimal amount of posterior acoustic shadowing (Fig. 3.21). The larger the haemangioma, the less characteristic are the features and the more difficult it is to differentiate the lesion from a large tumour.

Fibronodular hyperplasia

Discrete areas of fibronodular hyperplasia may be difficult to differentiate

Fig. 3.20 The exact size, number and location of multiple hepatic cysts may be determined by intraoperative or laparoscopic ultrasound during deroofing procedures. AE, acoustic enhancement.

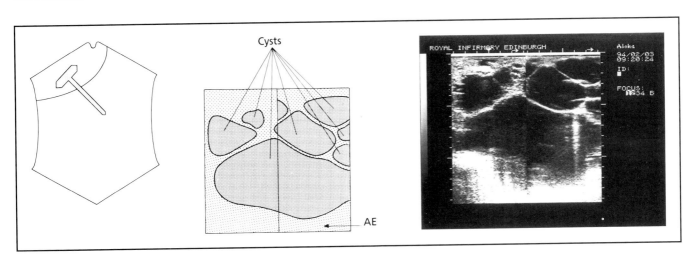

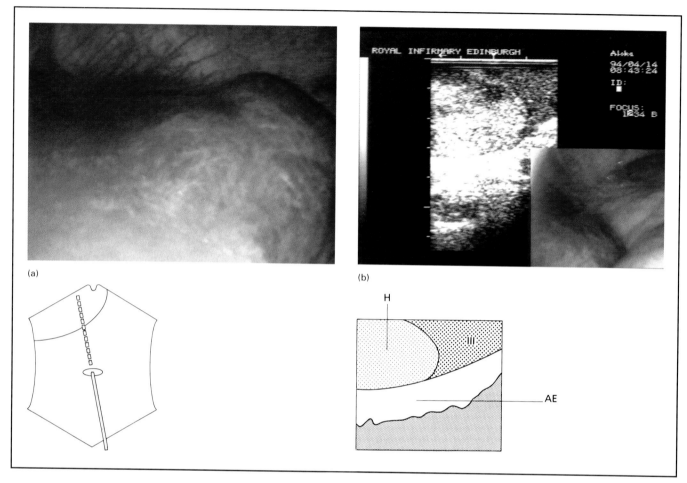

Fig. 3.21 (a) Laparoscopic inspection of the left hepatic lobe reveals a large mass lesion discovered incidentally during laparoscopic cholecystectomy. (b) Laparoscopic ultrasonography (7.5 MHz linear array) demonstrates features pathognomonic of a cavernous haemangioma. The lesion is hyperechoic compared with the surrounding normal hepatic parenchyma of segment III but with posterior acoustic enhancement. H, haemargioma; AE, acoustic enhancement.

from other neoplasms on ultrasound features alone, but often such lesions have a bright hyperechoic centre which is thought to be due to the central scarring or fibrosis in the tumour (Fig. 3.22). Targeted biopsy of such a lesion may be undertaken under intraoperative or laparoscopic guidance.

Adenoma

The diagnosis of such lesions is generally made preoperatively, but laparoscopic evaluation may help in defining the nature and location of such lesions in addition to facilitating targeted biopsy. Intraoperative ultrasonography is invaluable in the planning of resection of the tumour. The diagnosis can rarely be made on ultrasound features alone and such tumours are often difficult to differentiate from fibronodular hyperplasia as a result (Fig. 3.23).

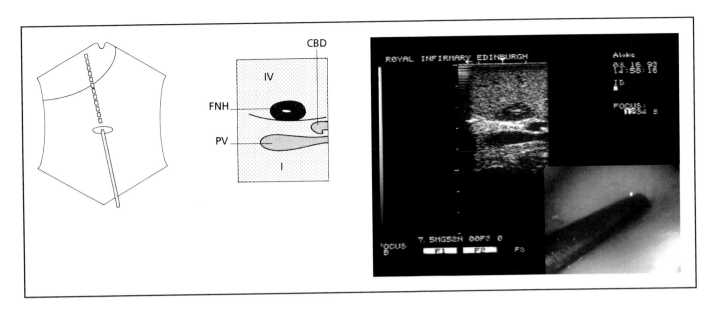

Fig. 3.22 Segment IV lesion discovered incidentally by laparoscopic ultrasonography during laparoscopic cholecystectomy in a 30-year-old woman taking an oral contraceptive. Its hypoechoic nature with a central hyperechoic scar characterises the lesion as fibronodular hyperplasia (FNH). CBD, common bile duct; PV, portal vein.

Other benign hepatic pathology

In the cirrhotic patient regenerating nodules may be difficult to differentiate from hepatoma. The instillation of saline into the abdominal cavity is particularly useful when examining the cirrhotic liver, since contact is maintained between the probe and the nodular surface of the liver. The liver parenchyma in such patients is generally hyperechoic and the degradation in the image may make it difficult to image anything other than a substantial tumour. None the less, discrete nodules can be submitted to definitive targeted biopsy.

Fatty infiltration of the liver results in increased acoustic impedance of the hepatic parenchyma. This abnormality is invariably uniform although, on occasion, a discrete area of fatty infiltration will mimic a hyperechoic tumour. In practical terms fatty infiltration will produce difficulties if there is a suspected hepatic lesion located deep in the liver. If increased echoity interferes with evaluation of a suspected hepatic lesion the total gain of the ultrasound machine may require to be adjusted and the near-field enhancement reduced.

Interpretation of the ultrasound image may be rendered difficult if there is associated pathology of the biliary tree. In the patient who has undergone previous stenting of the bile duct, sphincterotomy or surgical bypass, air in the biliary tree may produce considerable bright echoic lesions with posterior acoustic shadowing. Similarly, gross dilatation of the biliary tree in the jaundiced patient may hide small hepatic lesions.

Hepatoma

Primary hepatic tumours may appear as hyperechoic lesions with a surrounding echolucent rim (Fig. 3.24). They may, however, be difficult to define clearly in the cirrhotic patient and appear as isoechoic lesions with few internal echoes and no hypoechoic rim. Their presence may only be apparent by

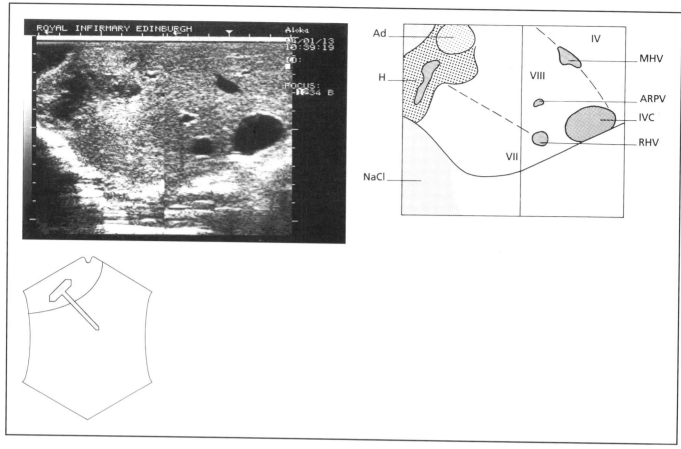

Fig. 3.23 A 25-year-old woman taking oral contraceptive presented with a spontaneous haemorrhage into the right liver associated with an underlying mass lesion. At laparotomy, intraoperative ultrasound was performed following full mobilisation of the right hemiliver. A well-defined hyperechoic lesion typical of an adenoma (Ad) was demonstrated within segment VIII, associated with extensive intrahepatic haematoma (H), which appeared heterogeneous and predominantly echopoor. A right hepatectomy was undertaken. ARPV, anterior sectoral branch of right portal vein; IVC, inferior vena cava; MHV, middle hepatic vein; NaCl, saline instillate; RHV, right hepatic vein.

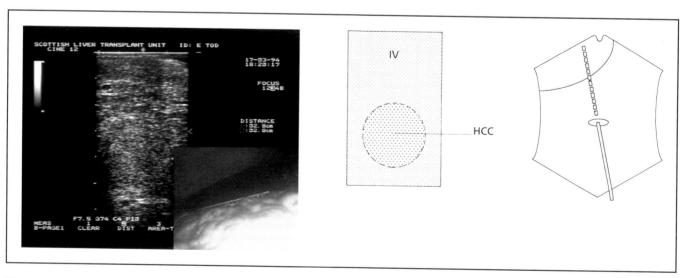

Fig. 3.24 Laparoscopic ultrasound in a patient with cirrhosis has defined a 2-cm hepatoma (HCC) with the same echo-texture as the surrounding diseased hepatic parenchyma. The demonstration of such isoechoic lesions is facilitated by dynamic real-time scanning.

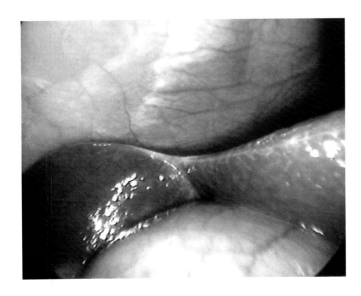

Fig. 3.25 Laparoscopic inspection of the liver in a patient with hepatocellular carcinoma revealed relative hypoperfusion of the left hemiliver reflecting left portal vein occlusion with tumour thrombus.

the distortion of the normal hepatic anatomy. Local dissemination of hepatoma is characteristically by the portal route and tumour thrombus may therefore be evident on ultrasound examination.

Operative ultrasonography is of immense value in the management of patients with primary hepatic malignancy [1,4,5]. Laparoscopy alone may be useful in detecting unsuspected cirrhosis, may reveal vascular invasion (Fig. 3.25) or may demonstrate peritoneal or overt hepatic dissemination of disease (Fig. 3.26) in patients with a preoperative diagnosis of hepatoma, but it is unlikely that any other than the most superficial of tumours will be visualised. The use of ultrasound during laparoscopy will localise any known tumour and demonstrate local invasiveness such as tumour thrombus extension into the adjacent portal venous branch (Fig. 3.27). The relationship of the tumour to the adjacent vessels can be determined and resectability judged on this information. It can be used to exclude the presence of other intrahepatic lesions, thereby avoiding an unnecessary and inappropriate

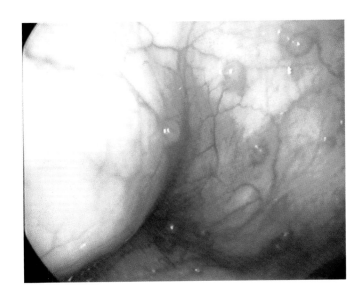

Fig. 3.26 Staging laparoscopy in a patient with hepatocellular carcinoma unexpectedly revealed multiple small peritoneal tumour seedlings.

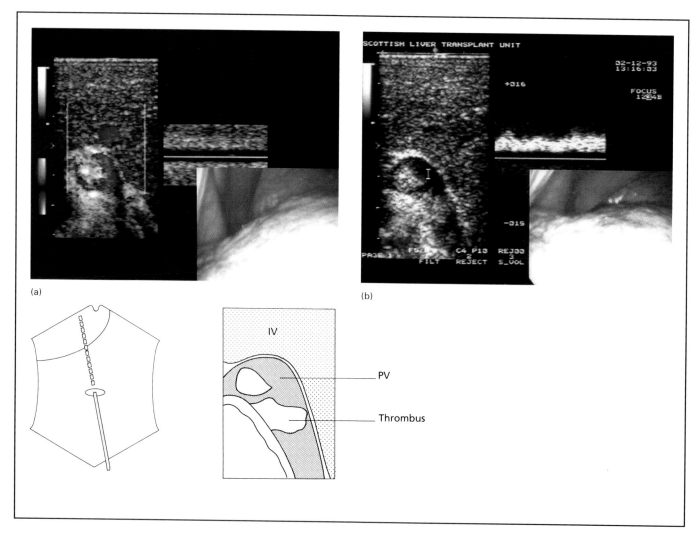

resection. Furthermore, placement of the probe at the porta hepatis and coeliac region may demonstrate lymph node enlargement or involvement by tumour.

In those patients submitted to laparotomy, intraoperative ultrasonography will provide additional information to that obtained from preoperative investigation. The examination is clearly not designed to replace preoperative radiological investigations but will provide additional information which will assist the surgeon in undertaking an appropriate resection. The operator can identify with ease the vascular structures from the portal venous branches to the hepatic veins as they run to the vena cava. When the lesion has been identified its relationship with the vessels can be established and its exact position determined.

Histological confirmation of the tumour can be established at the time of surgery by fine needle ultrasound guided biopsy or aspiration, and other suspicious areas in the liver can be similarly sampled. Since ultrasonography can assess the degree of vascular invasion, the extent of the hepatic resection can be determined. Techniques have been developed that can help to limit the extent of the resection. Using ultrasound guidance methylene blue dye

Fig. 3.27 (a) Laparoscopic sonogram demonstrating occlusion of the main portal vein (PV) with tumour thrombus. Doppler sampling revealed no detectable flow. The image is enhanced by colour Doppler flow imaging.
(b) Laparoscopic ultrasonography has defined invasion of PV with tumour thrombus. Doppler flow sampling confirms the absence of flow in the occluded vessel.

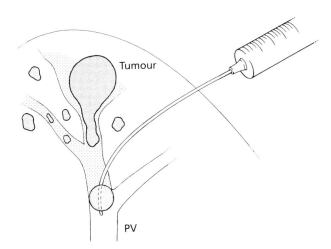

Fig. 3.28 Diagrammatic representation of tumour spread along the portal venous (PV) route and the use of a balloon catheter to facilitate segmental resection.

can be injected into the portal branch supplying the tumour to improve the definition of the segment or subsegment involved. By employing a Seldinger technique, a balloon catheter can be guided into the supplying segmental branch of the portal vein (Fig. 3.28). Haemostasis can be secured during segmental resection by inflating the balloon and occluding the right hepatic artery since such resections are more appropriate for tumours situated in the right hemiliver. The segment of the liver to be resected is demarcated clearly on the liver surface or with the aid of the injection of some dye proximal to the balloon. The excision of the tumour can be undertaken in a bloodless field with the minimal loss of functioning hepatic parenchyma.

In the surgery of primary liver tumours ultrasound is indispensable where the liver is the seat of an underlying cirrhosis [4,26]. In a series of 77 patients undergoing surgery for hepatoma and examined in this way [4], preoperative ultrasonography provided supplementary information in 33% of cases. In 21 of the 26 patients the intended surgical procedure was modified. In seven cases operative ultrasonography showed that the tumour was inoperable; on two occasions it demonstrated that a more radical resection was required and in the remaining 12 cases the lesion was sufficiently well localised by ultrasonography that a lesser resection was possible. In the same series of patients, 10 of the 30 resections were undertaken using the technique of ultrasonically guided injection of methylene blue dye or occlusion of portal segmental vessels [4].

These apparent technical advances have apparently been translated into long-term benefit. Lau *et al.* [27] observed a significant reduction in the rate of tumour involvement of the resection margin (0 versus 16%) when the results of operative ultrasound guided resection were compared to those from a historical control group.

Metastatic tumours

Metastases to the liver may arise from a primary tumour at any site in the body, but it is the colorectal metastasis which is of considerable interest to the hepatobiliary surgeon. Intraoperative ultrasonography may, however, be

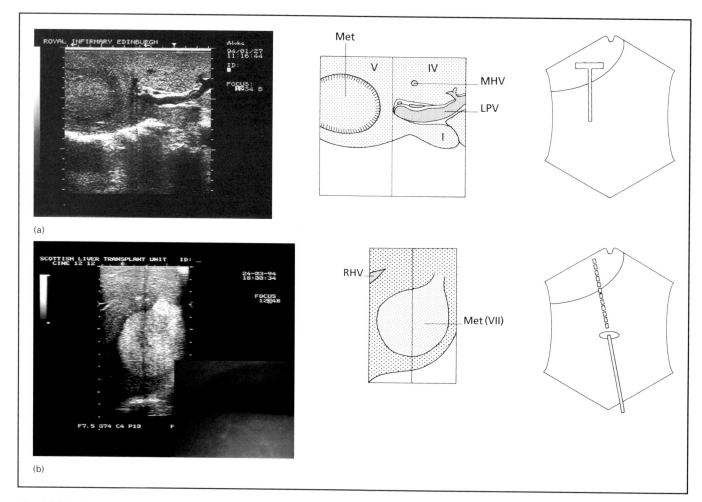

Fig. 3.29 (a) Intraoperative sonogram showing the typical 'bull's-eye' or target lesion appearance of a solitary 7-cm colorectal metastasis (Met) in the right hemiliver. The tumour was clear of the bifurcation of the portal vein and the middle hepatic vein (MHV), thus permitting resection by right hepatectomy. Note the portal venous branch to segment IV arising from the left portal vein (LPV). The left hepatic duct is just visible anteriorly. (b) A hyperechoic 6-cm solitary colorectal liver metastasis (Met) lying within hepatic segment VII has been defined during staging laparoscopic ultrasonography. RHV, right hepatic vein.

of value to the general surgeon, enabling detection of metastases to the liver at the time of apparently curative resection of the colorectal primary lesion [6,28–31]. For the hepatic surgeon operative ultrasonography is an indispensable tool in assessing the resectability of the metastasis [32]. The recent development of laparoscopic ultrasonography has now provided a useful means of evaluating patients referred for consideration of hepatic resection [11,12].

The ultrasound appearances of hepatic metastases are extremely variable and can be hyperechoic, hypoechoic or isoechoic in relation to the surrounding hepatic parenchyma. The tumour itself may be homogenous or heterogenous and the ultrasound image beyond the lesion may be unchanged,

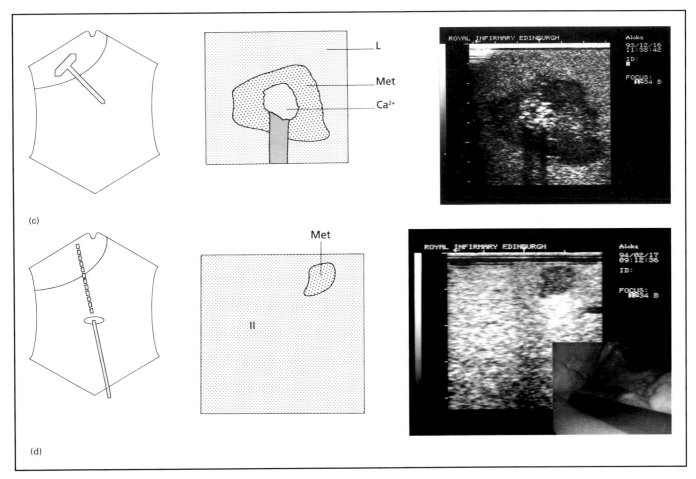

Fig. 3.29 (*Continued*) (c) A well-defined 6-cm colorectal liver metastasis (Met) detected by intraoperative ultrasound scanning. The lesion is hypoechoic compared with the surrounding liver parenchyma (L) and exhibits central dystrophic calcification (Ca^{2+}), which casts posterior acoustic shadows. (d) Laparoscopic sonogram demonstrating an 8-mm diameter hypoechoic metastasis (Met) within segment II of the left hepatic lobe. By contrast, the surrounding liver parenchyma is uniformly hyperechoic due to the fatty infiltration of alcoholic hepatitis. Note the umbilicated metastasis visible laparoscopically at the tip of the left hepatic lobe (insert).

absent, attenuated or increased. Colorectal metastasis are classically described as having a 'bull's-eye' appearance with a well-defined border, a hypoechoic rim and a hyperechoic centre (Fig. 3.29(a,b)). Larger lesions may have a densely hyperechoic central portion with posterior acoustic shadowing as a result of calcification within the lesion (Fig. 3.29(c)). Other tumours may have undergone cystic degeneration and a hypoechoic centre may be observed, but such lesions differ from benign hepatic cysts in exhibiting a well-defined hyperechoic wall. The isoechoic metastasis may be difficult to identify and may only be differentiated from normal liver by the subtle distortion or displacement of the intrahepatic vessels or by the presence of coexisting liver disease (Fig. 3.29(d)).

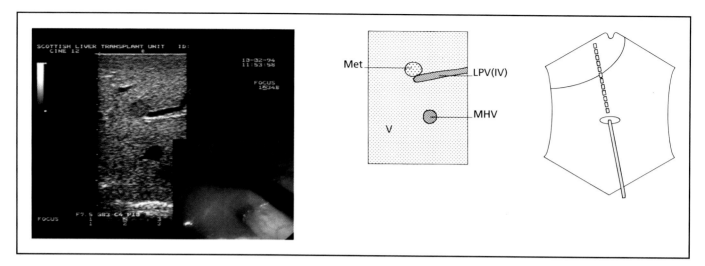

Metastases are more commonly found in the right lobe of the liver than the left side. In undertaking the examination of the liver it is often useful to characterise the nature of the lesion that is known to be present in the liver, so that a more educated search for other lesions can be undertaken. In this way it may be possible to identify tumours measuring as small as 5 mm in diameter, although this is dependent on the lesions echoity being different from that to the surrounding liver (Fig. 3.30). At laparotomy, intraoperative ultrasonography may provide more information than has been obtained from preoperative radiological investigation.

When the lesion has been identified, its relationship with the intrahepatic vessels can be established and its exact position determined from knowledge of the segmental anatomy of the liver (Fig. 3.31). Armed with this knowledge, the surgeon can assess the degree of vascular invasion and the extent of the hepatic resection can be determined (Fig. 3.32). The line of resection can be mapped out on the liver surface and ultrasound can be used to ensure that the planned line of resection is maintained.

Histological confirmation of the tumour can be established at the time of surgery by fine needle ultrasound guided biopsy and other suspicious areas in the liver can be similarly sampled (Fig. 3.33). Once the lesion to be biopsied has been imaged the angle of approach should be planned avoiding the portal tracts and the hepatic veins. The tip of the needle is scratched with a scalpel blade to increase the reflection from the ultrasound signal and so better identify the position of the tip of the needle during biopsy. Once it has passed into the lesion, the tip of the needle is seen as a bright hyperechoic image with posterior acoustic shadowing.

In the same way that intraoperative ultrasonography can be used to localise and facilitate biopsy of a lesion, so it can be used to target interstitial therapy. Ablation of tumour can be carried out by application of a diathermy current, by the instillation of absolute alcohol, by the insertion of cryotherapy probes [33,34] or by the direction of laser energy through a fibre into the tumour [35]. Of the various interstitial treatments, laser therapy is the modality that appears to provide a consistent area of tissue necrosis that can be readily monitored by intraoperative ultrasound (Fig. 3.34).

Fig. 3.30 Hypoechoic metastasis (Met) measuring less than 1 cm in diameter and lying adjacent to a segmental portal branch to IV (LPV(IV)) and the middle hepatic vein (MHV), detected by staging laparoscopic ultrasonography. This patient who had been thought preoperatively to have a solitary metastasis in the left lobe of the liver did not undergo resection.

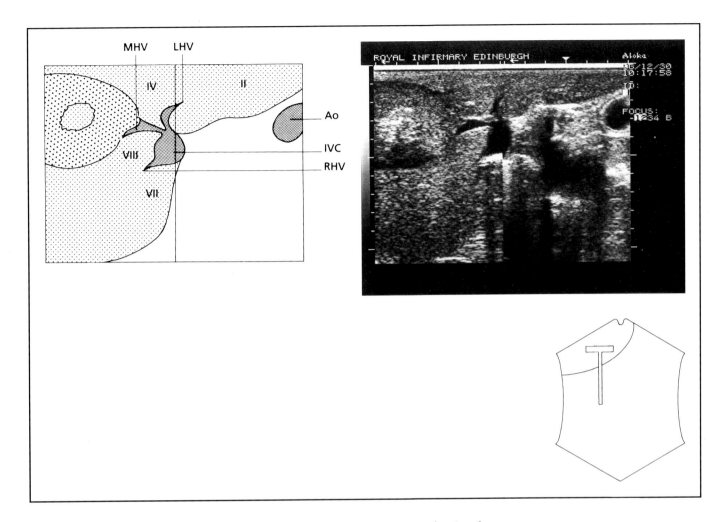

Fig. 3.31 Intraoperative sonogram showing a calcified colorectal metastasis situated centrally within the liver and obliterating the middle hepatic vein (MHV). Precise localisation of the right hepatic vein (RHV) using intraoperative ultrasound facilitated anatomical resection of segments IV, V and VIII. Ao, aorta; IVC, inferior vena cava; LHV, left hepatic vein.

Operative ultrasonography in the assessment of hepatic malignancy

Operative ultrasonography is likely to be of value in one of two situations. The hepatobiliary surgeon may require further information before proceeding to hepatic resection and the general surgeon may require accurate detection of hepatic involvement when undertaking resection of a primary gastrointestinal tumour.

Resectability of liver tumours

Early tumour recurrence following hepatic resection has been associated with the presence of extrahepatic tumour spread (including regional lymph node spread) and residual intrahepatic tumour which has not been recognised at the time of surgery. It is therefore essential for the surgeon to be aware of the size, site and number of hepatic tumours, in addition to their vascular relationships. Although a variety of preoperative investigations may provide some of this information, only operative ultrasonography can provide the surgeon with immediate information that facilitates hepatic resection along recognised anatomical planes (Fig. 3.35).

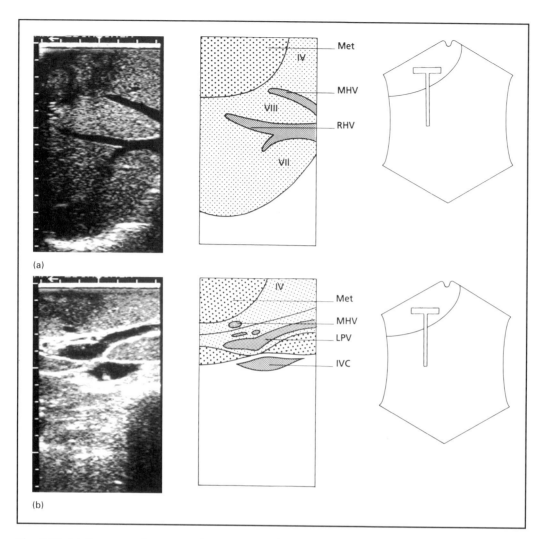

Fig. 3.32 (a) Transverse intraoperative sonogram obtained with the T-probe placed upon segment IV and angled cephalad through the liver identifying the hepatic venous confluence. The hypoechoic metastatic tumour (Met) encroaches across the functional midline of the liver identified by the middle hepatic vein (MHV). An extended right hepatectomy (resection of segments IV–VIII) was required to achieve complete resection. RHV, right hepatic vein. (b) Transverse IOUS with the probe in the same position as in Fig. 3.32(a) but angled more caudally. This manoeuvre achieves a transverse image of the porta hepatis. Note the proximity of the tumour (Met) to the portal venous bifurcation. IVC, inferior vena cava; LPV, left portal vein.

The value of intraoperative ultrasonography is often difficult to ascertain from enthusiastic surgical proponents of the technique. It may provide diagnostic information otherwise not available, may replace or complement preoperative radiography or guide surgical procedures [36]. Thus, Machi *et al.* [36] were able to report that beneficial information was obtained in 89% of hepatic operations and altered the previously planned surgical procedure in 32 of 82 such cases (39%). Clarke *et al.* [37] reported that operative ultrasonography detected additional lesions in 25 and 35% of examinations

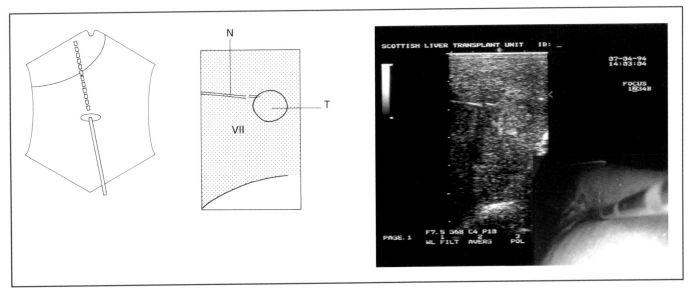

Fig. 3.33 Laparoscopic ultrasound guided needle biopsy of a hyperechoic 12-mm metastasis (T) in hepatic segment VII. The passage of the needle appears as a hyperechoic linear artefact (N) which may be accentuated by abrading the needle tip.

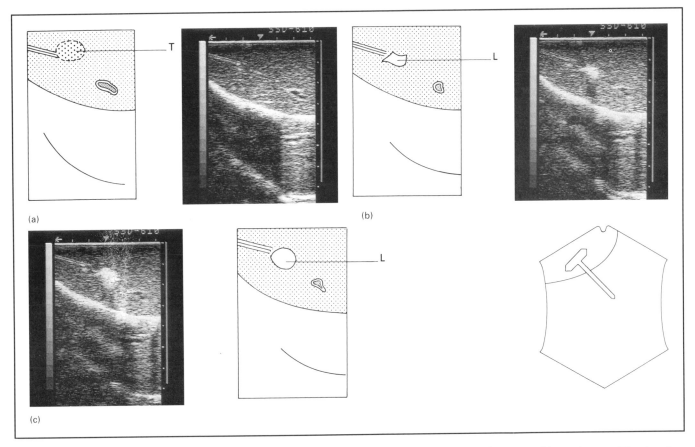

Fig. 3.34 Intraoperative ultrasound guidance of interstitial laser therapy. The tip of a Nd : YAG laser fibre has been introduced into a small hepatocellular carcinoma (T). Local tissue ablation is readily observed by the development of a slowly expanding hyperechoic lesion (L) with posterior acoustic shadowing.

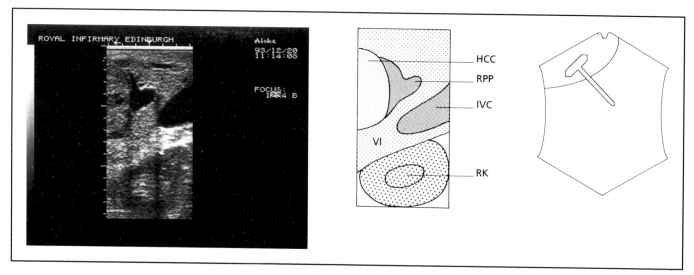

when compared to preoperative ultrasonography and dynamic computerised tomography (CT) scanning respectively in 54 patients with a variety of liver tumours. Forty per cent of the tumours were neither visible nor palpable at operation. Others [38] have reported a sensitivity rate for operative ultrasound of 98% compared to 77% for preoperative CT scanning in 45 patients with liver metastases. Soyer *et al.* [39] improved the sensitivity of dynamic CT scanning to 89% when this investigation was combined with transabdominal ultrasonography and CT angioportography, but this still fell short of the sensitivity rate of operative ultrasonography which detected 96% of hepatic lesions in the 37 patients studied.

Fig. 3.35 A large solitary hepatocellular carcinoma (HCC) situated astride the bifurcation of the right portal pedicle (RPP) was defined by intraoperative ultrasound assessment. Compensatory hypertrophy of the left hemiliver was sufficient to allow an extended right hepatectomy despite the underlying cirrhosis. IVC, inferior vena cava; RK, right kidney.

Detection of occult liver metastases

The importance of accurate staging of liver involvement by the primary tumour in determining outcome is well established. Finlay and McArdle [8,40] demonstrated that at least 20% of patients with colorectal carcinoma, and in whom an apparently curative resection had been undertaken, concealed occult hepatic metastases at the time of their initial surgery and that this was the single most important determinant of long-term survival. Intraoperative ultrasound scanning has been shown to be the most sensitive method for detecting these impalpable tumours. Charnley *et al.* [41] reported that operative ultrasonography diagnosed more metastases than palpation — abdominal ultrasonography or CT scanning in 99 patients undergoing surgery for colorectal cancer — identifying metastases in 24 of the 26 patients (91%) subsequently shown to have lesions. Others have confirmed that it is possible to detect lesions less than 10 mm in diameter and occult metastases have been demonstrated by operative ultrasound where both preoperative investigations and palpation of the liver have previously failed in up to 10% of laparotomies [30,37,42,43].

We have studied a group of patients undergoing resection of colonic malignancy to compare intraoperative ultrasonography with iodised oil-enhanced CT scanning in the detection of hepatic metastases. Of the 72 patients who underwent both procedures, 17 were reported to have metastases on CT scan. In only 13 of these patients did operative ultrasound scan confirm these findings and a further three patients who had metastases demonstrated by intraoperative ultrasound scan subsequently had lesions detected on follow-up CT scan. When a direct comparison was made between the two techniques it was observed that intraoperative ultrasound scanning (IOUS) detected 39 metastases compared to 29 metastases by CT scanning.

Laparoscopic ultrasonography in the assessment of hepatic malignancy

Our more recent experience with laparoscopy, augmented by laparoscopic ultrasound as a preoperative staging investigation in patients considered potential candidates for resection of their liver tumours, has demonstrated that a substantial proportion of unnecessary laparotomies can be avoided, and that at the very least, laparoscopic ultrasound complements existing investigations in improving patient selection for operation [10–12]. In our own experience, unnecessary laparotomy has rarely been undertaken when benign disease has masqueraded as malignancy. Just as intraoperative contact ultrasonography has improved the practice of resectional liver surgery, laparoscopic ultrasonography can be used to plan and modify the surgical approach to liver resection.

Our recent experience of 52 patients considered to have liver tumours potentially suitable for liver resection with curative intent have been reviewed [11]. The types of liver tumour ultimately confirmed following full investigation are shown in Table 3.1. Thirty-eight patients (73%) had undergone previous abdominal operations but abdominal adhesions prevented laparoscopy in only two cases (4% failure rate), and limited the examination to one side of the liver in a further two patients.

Laparoscopy identified the liver tumour in only 34 out of 50 patients (68%), and the presence of hepatic cirrhosis was diagnosed and confirmed with biopsy in six. The irresectable nature of the known hepatic malignancy was demonstrated during laparoscopy in 23 patients (46%). Extrahepatic tumour spread was identified in 18 cases and bilobar dissemination of disease was demonstrated in 11 patients. In four cases, primary extrahepatic tumour sites were discovered in patients thought to have primary hepatic malignancy, but shown to have irresectable hepatic metastases (caecum, gall bladder, pancreas and stomach, respectively). Laparotomy was avoided in all but the first, in whom a palliative right hemicolectomy was undertaken. In two patients with histologically confirmed irresectable liver secondaries the source of the primary tumour was not determined.

Laparoscopic ultrasound was not performed in seven of the 50 patients assessed laparoscopically (14%), since laparoscopy alone had already

Type	Tumour	Number	Per cent
Primary (n = 9)	Hepatocellular carcinoma	8	15
	Cholangiocarcinoma	1	2
Secondary (n = 37)	Colorectal	28	54
	Ovarian	1	2
	Cervix	1	2
	Gallbladder	1	2
	Stomach	1	2
	Pancreas	1	2
	Gastric leiomyosarcoma	1	2
	Colonic leiomyosarcoma	1	2
	Unknown primary	2	4
Non-malignant (n = 6)	Focal nodular hyperplasia	2	4
	Cavernous haemangioma	1	2
	Regenerating nodule	1	2
	Fibrous tissue	1	2
	Simple cyst	1	2

Table 3.1 Underlying hepatic pathology in 52 patients assessed for resectability of suspected hepatic neoplasia by laparoscopic ultrasonography from 1991 to 1993

provided sufficient information to indicate that surgical resection was inappropriate. In 14 of the remaining 43 patients (33%), laparoscopic ultrasonography demonstrated liver tumours which had not been visible on laparoscopic inspection.

Further information regarding tumour resectability was obtained in 18 of 43 patients (42%) and included demonstration of bilobar liver disease in 14 cases, hilar lymphadenopathy in five patients and portal or hepatic venous invasion in five instances. Seven of the 43 patients (16%) were shown by laparoscopic ultrasonography alone to have irresectable disease, when preceding investigations (including laparoscopy) had demonstrated no contraindication to operation. The management of two further patients, thought on presentation to have hepatic malignancy, was modified as a direct result of the laparoscopic ultrasound examination. A regenerating cirrhotic nodule was confirmed by laparoscopic ultrasound with guided biopsy in a patient originally considered as having a small hepatoma within a cirrhotic liver. The second patient, presenting 2 years after resection of a carcinoma of the sigmoid colon, was thought to have a colorectal liver metastasis, having declared with rising serum carcinoembryonic antigen levels and a small CT detected lesion within the right liver. Laparoscopic ultrasound indicated this lesion to be a simple cyst, a finding supported by a follow-up CT scan 6 months later. Thus, additional information derived exclusively from the ultrasound component of the laparoscopic examination directly affected patient management in nine cases.

Factors precluding attempts at liver resection were demonstrated in four patients in whom laparoscopic and laparoscopic ultrasound staging had indicated no contraindication to liver resection. Pulmonary metastases which

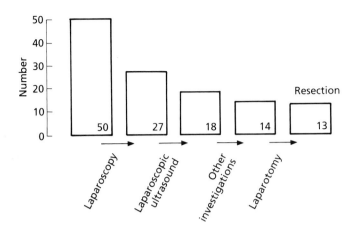

Fig. 3.36 Reduction in patients submitted to laparotomy as a consequence of the introduction of laparoscopy and laparoscopic ultrasonography in the assessment of hepatic malignancy. See text for explanation of groups. (After John *et al.* [11], with permission.)

had been missed by chest X-ray were defined by thoracic CT scans in three cases, and sequential computed tomography angioportography (CTAP) examinations indicated irresectable bilobar liver deposits in three patients. These represent the only known false-negative laparoscopic ultrasound examinations in this series.

The impact of laparoscopy with laparoscopic ultrasonography upon the selection of patients for operative assessment and liver resection is shown in Fig. 3.36. Fourteen (28%) of the 50 patients who underwent laparoscopic evaluation were ultimately assessed by laparotomy, in 13 (93%) of whom liver resection with curative intent was undertaken. A benign nodule of fibrous connective tissue at the root of the falciform ligament and thought to be a colorectal liver metastasis at laparoscopy, was finally confirmed at laparotomy with open biopsy in the one patient who did not undergo liver resection following abdominal exploration. This non-therapeutic laparotomy following a false-positive staging laparoscopy represents the only such example in this series.

The introduction of laparoscopic staging has had a major impact on our hepatic surgical practice. Thirty-eight patients with malignant liver tumours underwent exploratory laparotomy and operative assessment of resectability

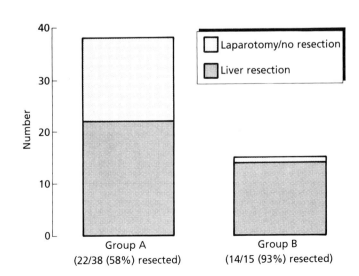

Fig. 3.37 Impact of laparoscopy and laparoscopic ultrasonography on the selection of patients with suspected hepatic malignancy for operative assessment and liver resection. (After John *et al.* [11], with permission.)

before staging with laparoscopy and laparoscopic ultrasound was routinely performed in our own unit (group A), with only 15 patients managed in this way following the adoption of this procedure (group B) (Fig. 3.37). It is accepted that variables other than the adoption of laparoscopic staging may have contributed to these changes in practice. Nevertheless, the high proportion of patients in this series who displayed overt, albeit unsuspected, extrahepatic tumour spread within the abdomen at laparoscopy makes a strong case in favour of staging laparoscopy prior to planned operative assessment of resectability of liver malignancies. Furthermore, the incorporation of laparoscopy and ultrasonography into the investigative algorithm of such patients seems appropriate as the most sensitive method for detecting local and regional dissemination of tumour.

References

1 Garden OJ. Operative ultrasonography. *Hospital Update* 1992; 18: 470–9.
2 Fortner JG, Maclean BJ, Kim DK, *et al*. The seventies evolution in liver surgery for cancer. *Cancer* 1981; 47: 2162–6.
3 Adson MA. Resection of liver metastases — when is it worthwhile? *World J Surg* 1987; 11: 511–20.
4 Bismuth H, Castaing D, Garden OJ. The use of operative ultrasound in surgery of primary liver tumours. *World J Surg* 1987; 11: 610–14.
5 Makuuchi M, Hasegwa H, Yamazaki S, Takayasu K, Moriyama N. The use of operative ultrasound as an aid to liver resection in patients with hepatocellular carcinoma. *World J Surg* 1987; 11: 615–21.
6 Castaing D, Emond J, Kunstlinger F, Bismuth H. Utility of operative ultrasound in the surgical management of liver tumors. *Ann Surg* 1986; 204: 600–5.
7 Goligher JC. The operability of carcinoma of the rectum. *Br Med J* 1941; ii: 393–7.
8 Finlay IG, McArdle CS. Effect of occult hepatic metastases on survival after curative resection for colorectal carcinoma. *Gastroenterology* 1983; 85: 596–9.
9 Harbin WP, Wittenberg J, Ferrucci JT, Mueller PR, Ottinger LW. Fallibility of exploratory laparotomy in detection of hepatic and retroperitoneal masses. *Am J Roentgenol* 1980; 135: 115–21.
10 John TG, Garden OJ. Laparoscopic ultrasonography for staging of abdominal malignancy. In: Garden OJ, Paterson-Brown S, eds. *Principles and Practice of Surgical Laparoscopy*. London: WB Saunders, 1994: 565–83.
11 John TG, Greig JD, Crosbie JL, Miles WFA, Garden OJ. Superior staging of liver tumours with laparoscopy and laparoscopic ultrasound. *Ann Surg* 1994 (in press).
12 John TG, Garden OJ. Laparoscopic ultrasound: extending the scope of diagnostic laparoscopy. *Br J Surg* 1994; 81: 5–6.
13 Windsor JA, Garden OJ. Laparoscopic ultrasonography. *Aust NZ J Surg* 1993; 63: 1–2.
14 Cuschieri A. Laparoscopy in diagnosis and staging of patients with cancer of the exocrine pancreas. In: Preece PE, Cuschieri A, Rosin RD, eds. *Cancer of the Bile Ducts and Pancreas*. Philadelphia: WB Saunders, 1989: 189–96.
15 Cuschieri A. Laparoscopy for pancreatic cancer: does it benefit the patient? *Eur J Surg Oncol* 1988; 14: 41–4.
16 Cuschieri A, Hall AW, Clark J. Value of laparoscopy in the diagnosis and management of pancreatic carcinoma. *Gut* 1978; 19: 672–7.
17 Warshaw AL, Gu ZY, Wittenberg J, Waltman AC. Preoperative staging and assessment of resectability of pancreatic cancer. *Arch Surg* 1990; 125: 230–3.

18 Lightdale CJ. Laparoscopy and biopsy in malignant liver disease. *Cancer* 1982; 50: 267–5

19 Jeffers L, Spieglman G, Reddy R, *et al*. Laparoscopically directed fine needle aspiration for the diagnosis of hepatocellular carcinoma: a safe and accurate technique. *Gastrointest Endosc* 1988; 34: 235–7.

20 Miles WFA, Paterson-Brown S, Garden OJ. Laparsocopic contact hepatic ultrasonography. *Br J Surg* 1992; 79: 419–20.

21 Bismuth H. Surgical anatomy and anatomical surgery of the liver. *World J Surg* 1982; 6: 3–9.

22 Couinaud C. *Le Foie Etudes Anatomiques et Chirurgicales*. Paris: Masson, 1957.

23 Makuuchi M, Hasegawa H, Yamasaki S, *et al*. Four new hepatectomy procedures for resection of the right hepatic vein and preservation of the inferior right hepatic vein. *Surg Gyn Obst* 1987; 164: 69–72.

24 Makuuchi M, Hasegawa H, Yamazaki S, *et al*. The inferior right hepatic vein: ultrasonic demonstration. *Radiology* 1983; 148: 213–17.

25 Mårvik R, Myrvold HE, Johnsen G, Røysland P. Laparoscopic ultrasonography and treatment of hepatic cysts. *Surg Laparosc Endosc* 1993; 3: 172–4.

26 Sheu J-C, Lee C-S, Sung J-L, Chen D-S, Yang P-M, Lin T-Y. Intraoperative hepatic ultrasonography—an indispensable procedure in resection of small hepatocellular carcinomas. *Surgery* 1985; 97: 97–103.

27 Lau WY, Leung KL, Lee TW, Li AKC. Ultrasonography during liver resection for hepatocellular carcinoma. *Br J Surg* 1993; 80: 493–4.

28 Charnley RM, Morris DL, Dennison AR, Amar SS, Hardcastle JD. Detection of colorectal liver metastases using intraoperative ultrasonography. *Br J Surg* 1991; 78: 45–8.

29 Machi J, Isomoto H, Yamashita Y, Kurohiji T, Shirouzu K, Kakegawa T. Intraoperative ultrasonography in screening for liver metastases from colorectal cancer: comparative accuracy with traditional procedures. *Surgery* 1987; 101: 678–84.

30 Stadler J, Hölscher AH, Adolf J. Intraoperative ultrasonographic detection of occult liver metastases in colorectal cancer. *Surg Endosc* 1991; 5: 36–40.

31 Stewart PJ, Chu JM, Kos SC, Chapuis PH, Bokey EL. Intra-operative ultrasound for the detection of hepatic metastases from colorectal cancer. *Aust NZ J Surg* 1993; 63: 530–4.

32 Gozzetti G, Mazziotti A, Bolondi L, *et al*. Intraoperative ultrasonography in surgery for liver tumours. *Surgery* 1986; 99: 523–9.

33 Onik G, Kane R, Steele G, *et al*. Monitoring hepatic cryosurgery with sonography. *Am J Roentgenol* 1986; 147: 665–9.

34 Ravikumar TS, Kane R, Cady B, *et al*. Hepatic cryosurgery with intraoperative ultrasound monitoring for metastatic colon carcinoma. *Arch Surg* 1987; 122: 403–9.

35 Schneider PD. Liver resection and laser hyperthermia. *Surg Clin Am* 1992; 72: 623–39.

36 Machi J, Sigel B, Zaren HA, Kurohiji T, Yamashita Y. Operative ultrasonography during hepatobiliary and pancreatic surgery. *World J Surg* 1993; 17: 640–6.

37 Clarke MP, Kane RA, Steele G Jr, *et al*. Prospective comparison of preoperative imaging and intraoperative ultrasonography in the detection of liver tumours. *Surgery* 1989; 106: 849–55.

38 Parker GA, Lawrence W, Horsley SJ, *et al*. Intraoperative ultrasound of the liver affects operative decision making. *Ann Surg* 1989; 209: 569–77.

39 Soyer P, Elias D, Zeitoun G, Roche A, Levesque M. Surgical treatment of hepatic metastases: impact of intraoperative sonography. *Am J Roentgenol* 1993; 160: 511–14.

40 Finlay IG, McArdle CS. Occult hepatic metastases in colorectal carcinoma. *Br J Surg* 1986; 73: 732–5.

41 Charnley RM, Morris DL, Dennison AR, Amar SS, Hardcastle JD. The detection of colorectal liver metastases using intraoperative ultrasound. *Br J Radiol* 1989.

42 Charnley RM, Hardcastle JD. Intraoperative abdominal ultrasound. *Gut* 1990; 31: 368–9.

43 Machi J, Isomoto H, Kurohiji T, *et al.* Accuracy of intraoperative ultrasound in diagnosing liver metastasis from colorectal cancer: evaluation with postoperative follow-up results. *World J Surg* 1991; 15: 551–7.

4: Intraoperative and Laparoscopic Ultrasound of the Pancreas

Introduction

The assessment of patients presenting with pancreatic carcinoma is directed at the establishment of a diagnosis, the accurate staging of disease and the evaluation of resectability in the small group of individuals in whom there is a prospect of cure [1]. Unfortunately, for the vast majority of patients the disease is often advanced at the time of diagnosis with there being early dissemination to peritoneum, lymph nodes and adjacent vessels. Despite the availability of abdominal ultrasonography, computerised tomography (CT), visceral angiography and, more recently, nuclear magnetic resonance imaging, no single investigation alone is able to satisfactorily assess tumour dissemination and determine local resectability with reasonable reliability.

Notwithstanding the considerable enthusiasm for the use of intraoperative ultrasonography in the assessment of hepatobiliary disease over recent years, surgeons have shown more restraint in taking up this form of operative investigation in the management of pancreatic disease. The fact that the pancreas lends itself well to intraoperative ultrasound evaluation is not in doubt, but pancreatic surgeons have tended to favour palpation of the gland, the use of wide exploration of the retroperitoneal area and trial dissection of the surrounding structures to assess resectability of pancreatic lesions at open surgery. None the less, a number of ultrasound enthusiasts have continued to champion the technique over the years in the evaluation of both neoplastic and inflammatory disease without perhaps convincing surgical colleagues that such imagery could be translated into a tangible benefit to the patient [2–5].

The arrival of laparoscopic ultrasonography may serve as the catalyst to remove the doubts of the sceptical surgeon that ultrasound has a role in the management of pancreatic disease. For suspected ampullary and pancreatic malignancy, intraoperative ultrasonography can be used to locate the lesion and assess the degree of local and more distant dissemination of disease, and for islet cell tumours ultrasound can localise small lesions which are impalpable at laparotomy. Laparoscopy has been recognised by a small band of enthusiasts as a useful means of assessing dissemination in pancreatic carcinoma, although it has a limited ability to detect anything other than overt spread of disease [6,7]. Now that identical ultrasound images can be obtained at laparoscopy there is a possibility of obtaining accurate detail of pancreatic pathology without having to submit the patient to open surgery [8–12].

This chapter will describe the intraoperative and laparoscopic ultrasound examination of the pancreas and highlight the areas where it it most likely to prove of clinical benefit.

Anatomy

The pancreas lies transversely in the retroperitoneum with its head situated to the right of the second lumbar vertebra and its tail reaching the splenic hilum at the level of the twelfth thoracic vertebra. Its anterior surface is covered by the peritoneum of the lesser sac. The head is encircled by the duodenum and is the thickest part of the gland, measuring approximately 3.5 cm in anteroposterior diameter. The neck of the gland is formed as it passes over the portal and superior mesenteric veins in the midline and is the thinnest part of the pancreas, measuring only 1.5 cm in anteroposterior diameter. The body and tail are separated from the stomach by the lesser sac and pass over the aorta with the splenic artery and vein running behind the gland (Fig. 4.1).

The hilum of the left kidney, the inferior vena cava and the left renal vein lie behind the head of the gland, whilst the uncinate process extends behind the superior mesenteric vein to reach the accompanying superior mesenteric artery. The coeliac trunk gives off the common hepatic artery to the right and the splenic artery to the left from their origin just superior to the neck of the gland. The superior mesenteric vein and artery emerge from beneath the lower border of the neck. The posterior surface of the body runs from in front of the aorta, the left adrenal gland, and the left renal vessels to the upper pole of the left kidney. The splenic artery runs a tortuous course along its upper border, whilst the accompanying vein is firmly embedded in the posterior surface of the gland.

The arterial blood supply of the pancreas is not often seen on preoperative radiological investigation, but operative ultrasound imaging may demonstrate the anterior and posterior pancreaticoduodenal arteries as they arise from the gastroduodenal artery. The anterior and posterior inferior pancreaticoduodenal arteries arise from the superior mesenteric artery and form anterior and posterior arcades with the vessels from the gastroduodenal artery.

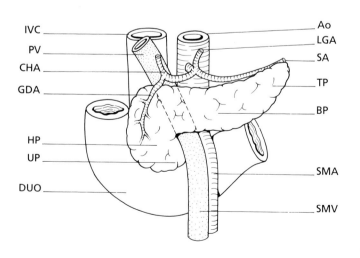

Fig. 4.1 Diagram of the pancreas and its relationship with the peripancreatic vasculature. Ao, aorta; BP, body of pancreas; CHA, common hepatic artery proper; DUO, duodenum; GDA, gastroduodenal artery; HP, head of pancreas; IVC, inferior vena cava; LGA, left gastric artery; PV, portal vein; SA, splenic artery; SMA, superior mesenteric artery; SMV, superior mesenteric vein; TP, tail of pancreas; UP, uncinate process of pancreas.

Ultrasound of the normal pancreas

The pancreas can be evaluated with either a linear-array or sectoral probe. The advantages and disadvantages of the two types of probe are not dissimilar to those which apply to examination of the liver. It is generally easier for the surgeon at open operation to employ a linear-array ultrasound probe which can be placed flat on the stomach and duodenum or the pancreas itself if some preliminary dissection has been undertaken. A T-shaped or I-shaped 5- or 7.5-MHz linear-array probe is generally employed at open surgery and the evaluation of the pancreas using this instrument will be described later. A 5-MHz transducer will provide considerable detail of the pancreas, although we have favoured the use of a 7.5-mHz linear-array transducer at laparoscopy [8,10]. Other workers have preferred to employ curvilinear-array probes with small convex transducer footprints which require only a small cross-sectional area of contact [13,14].

Intraoperative ultrasonography

The pancreas can be scanned through the left lobe of the liver, the stomach, the gastrocolic ligament or the transverse mesocolon before any dissection has been undertaken (Fig. 4.2). However, the best images may be obtained

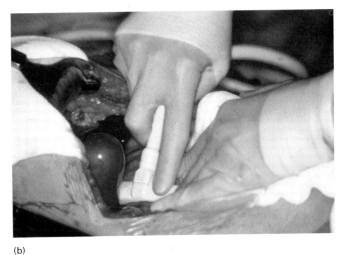

(b)

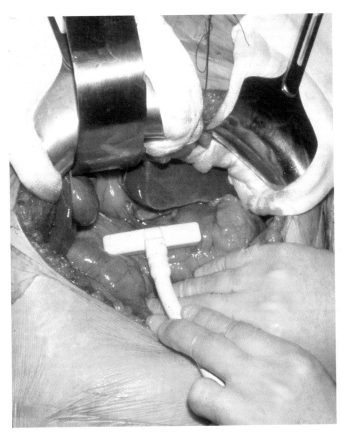

(a)

Fig. 4.2 T-shaped linear-array probe (5 MHz) applied to the stomach and transverse mesocolon in order to scan the pancreas at open operation. Both transverse scans in the long axis of the gland (a), and sagitally orientated scans giving cross-sectional cuts of the pancreas (b) may be obtained.

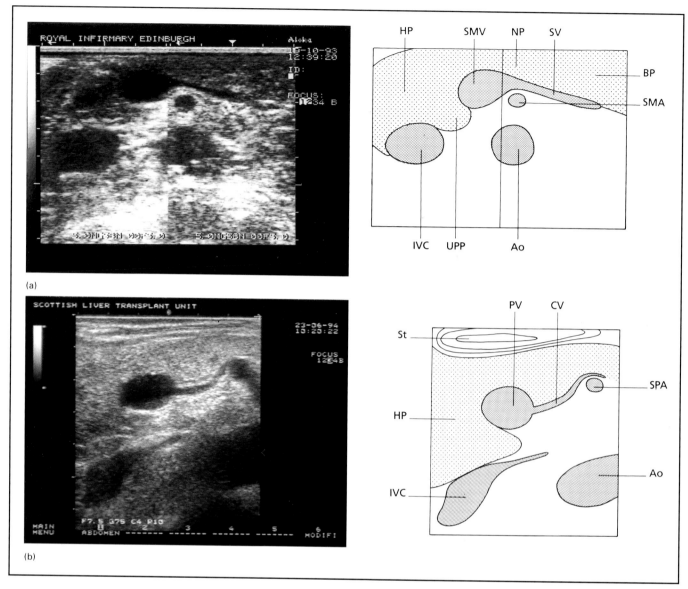

Fig. 4.3 (a) Transverse intraoperative sonograms of the pancreas obtained with a 7.5-MHz T-probe placed upon the gastric antrum (St). The head (HP), neck (NP) and body (BP) of the gland are demonstrated lying anterior to the abdominal aorta (Ao) and inferior vena cava (IVC). A low magnification cut at an inferior level demonstrates the superior mesenteric artery (SMA) and the confluence of the superior mesenteric vein (SMV) and splenic vein (SV) posterior to the NP. (b) Scanning at a more cranial level identifies the portal vein (PV) and its foregut tributaries and the major branches of the coeliac axis.

by direct apposition of the transducer with the surface of the pancreas after full exposure of the gland. The pancreas should be examined from head to tail with the probe placed in both longitudinal and transverse planes. It is not always necessary to supplement contact scanning by using a stand-off with saline solution in the abdominal cavity, but this may occasionally facilitate transducer contact and near-field scanning of the superficial surface of the gland.

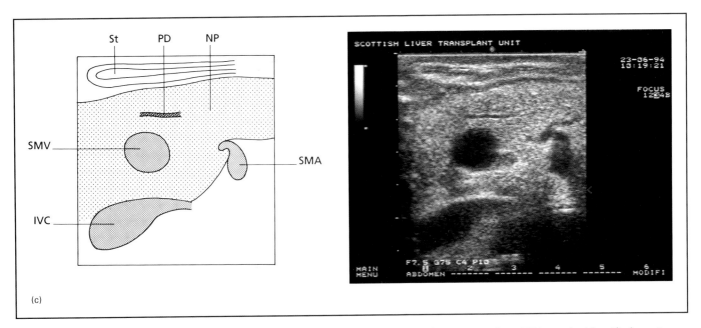

Fig. 4.3 (*Continued*) (c) The normal pancreatic duct (PD) may be identified passing within the pancreatic parenchyma at higher magnifications. Note how the uncinate process (UPP) of the pancreas extends to the left behind the SMV. CV, coronary vein; SPA, splenic artery. The probe position used in (a–c) is the same as that used in Fig. 4.10(a).

The examination of the pancreas commences with the linear-array probe placed transversely over the head of the gland (i.e. in the long axis of the pancreas) (Fig. 4.2(a)). The vena cava will be identified posteriorly and can be easily compressed if excessive pressure is applied. The vertical channel formed by the portal vein and superior mesenteric vein lies directly underneath the probe and is easily identified in cross-section behind the neck of the pancreas. The pancreatic duct may be seen in longitudinal and oblique cuts passing through the body, neck and head of the gland, although normally rarely exceeds 3 mm in diameter. At a slightly more caudal level the confluence of the superior mesenteric and splenic veins can be defined posterior to the neck of the pancreas, and the relationship of these structures with the uncinate process established. The superior mesenteric artery will be seen to arise from the aorta and run inferiorly on the left side of the superior mesenteric vein (Fig. 4.3).

The probe is displaced to the left to examine the body and tail of the gland. If this examination has been undertaken without full exposure of the gland it may be necessary to compress the stomach, which is interposed between the probe and the pancreas, to displace any stomach gas which might cause acoustic interference. The coeliac trunk and the origin of the common hepatic and splenic arteries can be followed distally as they emerge at the superior border of the gland. Para-aortic lymphadenopathy can be identified at this stage. As the probe is displaced towards the pancreatic tail the normal pancreatic duct becomes more attenuated and is often lost within the pancreatic parenchyma.

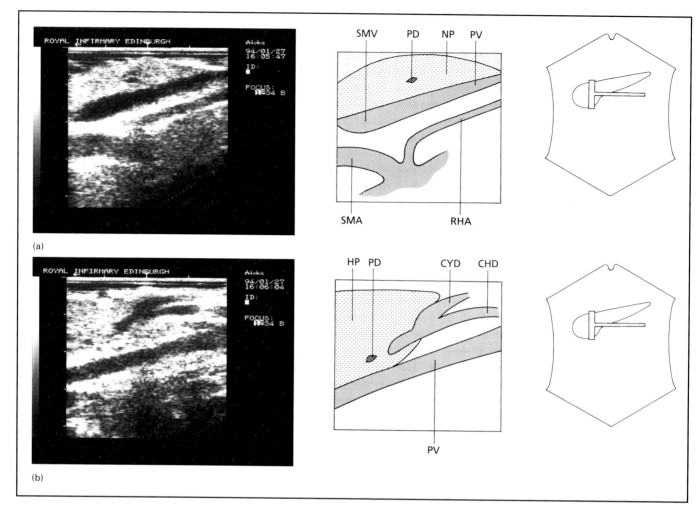

Fig. 4.4 (a) Parasagittal intraoperative sonograms of the pancreas with a 7.5-MHz T-probe placed upon the normal head (HP) and neck (NP) of the pancreas. The long axis of the superior mesenteric–portal venous trunk (SMV, PV) is identified passing immediately behind the narrow neck of the gland, within which the non-dilated pancreatic duct (PD) is identified in cross-section. The slightly oblique direction of this sonogram demonstrates the parallel course of the superior mesenteric artery (SMA) from which an aberrant right hepatic artery (RHA) is seen passing in a cranial direction posterior to the portal vein. (b) Angulation of the probe to the right identifies the divergent retropancreatic course of the common bile duct which is formed by the confluence of the common hepatic (CHD) and cystic duct (CYD) at the superior pancreatic border.

The examination of the pancreas is completed by scanning the organ with the probe in a sagittal/oblique orientation (see Fig. 4.2(b)), which provides cross-sectional images of the pancreas and defines the relationships of any pancreatic lesion with respect to the long axis of the major vessels lying posteriorly (Fig. 4.4). Similarly, the presence of lymphadenopathy and the patency of these vessels can be established.

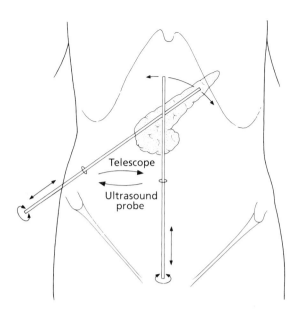

Fig. 4.5 Position of the laparoscopic ports for evaluation of the pancreas. Sagittal/oblique cuts obtained with the probe inserted through the umbilical port provide cross-sectional scans of the pancreas, whereas scanning from the right lateral port in a transverse/oblique direction provides images orientated about the long axis of the gland.

Laparoscopic ultrasonography

Laparoscopic ultrasound examination of the pancreas is performed under general anaesthesia by a standardised technique which is similar to that employed for laparoscopic evaluation of the liver using a 9-mm diameter linear-array contact ultrasound probe. Two disposable 10/11-mm laparoscopic cannulae are inserted at the umbilicus and right flank, and a thorough inspection of the abdominal cavity is performed using a 30° telescope. Particular attention is paid to evidence of metastatic disease involving the liver, mesenteric and hilar lymph nodes and all visible serosal surfaces. The techniques of supragastric bursoscopy and infragastric pancreoscopy are considered unnecessary, and no attempt is made to enter the lesser sac in order to visualise the pancreas directly. Placement of the ports in this configuration allows full examination of the pancreas in both cross-sectional and longitudinal planes using a rigid laparoscopic ultrasound probe (Fig. 4.5).

The liver is examined for evidence of metastatic disease and the presence of intrahepatic duct dilatation or pneumobilia, associated with distal biliary obstruction, and its relief by endoscopic sphincterotomy or biliary stent insertion noted (see Chapter 3). The hilar region should be examined for lymphadenopathy with the probe on the diaphragmatic surface of the liver (see Chapter 3). The probe is moved on to the hepatoduodenal ligament and the structures passing in the hepatic pedicle identified (see Chapter 2). The portal vein and common duct are easily recognised landmarks, and their distal retropancreatic course serves to guide the examination of the pancreas.

It is our own preference to commence the examination of the pancreas with the probe positioned in the umbilical port and the laparoscope in the right lumbar port. The portal vein is identified passing posterior to the neck of the pancreas, from which position of reference displacement or slight

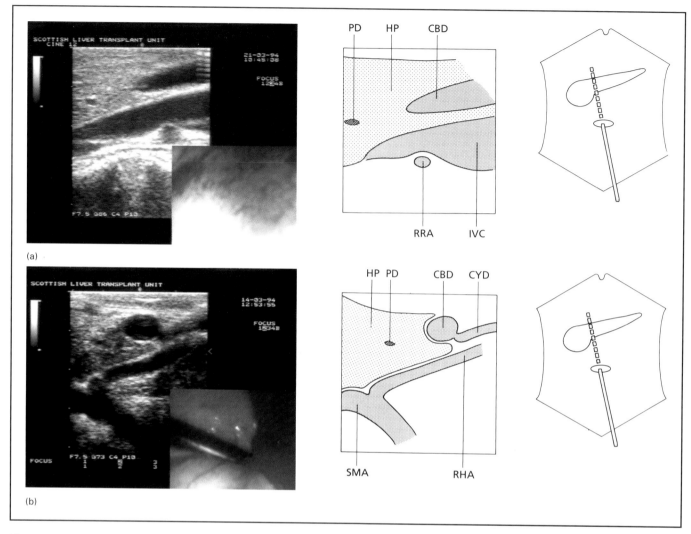

Fig. 4.6 (a) Parasagittal laparoscopic sonograms of the pancreas with a linear-array 7.5-MHz transducer placed upon the normal head of the pancreas (HP). The convergent courses of the pancreatic duct (PD) and common bile duct (CBD) are identified. The inferior vena cava (IVC) is recognised by its transmitted cardiac pulsation behind the HP at the level of the right renal artery (RRA).
(b) Angulation of the scanning direction more obliquely to the left identifies the superior mesenteric artery (SMA). An aberrant right hepatic artery (RHA) passing posterior to the HP and portal vein is readily identified from this position. CYD, cystic duct.

rotation of the transducer to the right identifies the head of the gland, whereas scanning to the left demonstrates the distal pancreatic parenchyma. Gradual clockwise rotation of the probe demonstrates the distal course of the common bile duct through or behind the head of the pancreas in progressively more oblique and cross-sectional cuts as it converges with the pancreatic duct towards the papilla of Vater (Fig. 4.6).

As the transducer is swept to the left, a cross-sectional image of the pancreatic body and tail can be examined throughout the length of the gland to its termination at the splenic hilum (Fig. 4.7).

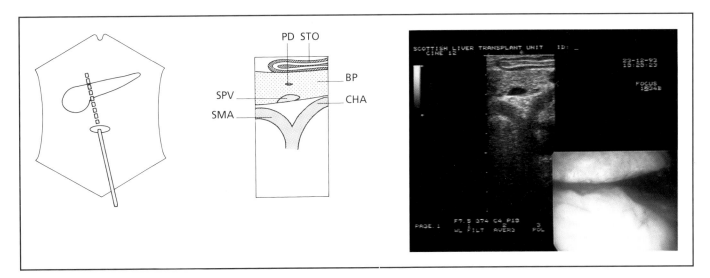

Fig. 4.7 Displacement of the laparoscopic ultrasound probe to the left provides cross-sectional images of the pancreatic body (BP) behind the stomach (STO). Slight angulation of the probe to the right has identified a common aortic origin for the superior mesenteric artery (SMA) and common hepatic artery (CHA) posteriorly. PD, pancreatic duct; SPV, splenic vein.

Reversal of camera and ultrasound probe positions, such that the transducer is manipulated from the right lateral port and placed upon the stomach, allows examination of the pancreas along its length (see Fig. 4.5). The splenic vein will be seen running along the posterior surface of the gland to its confluence with the superior mesenteric vein, although the splenic artery may not easily be visualised because of its tortuous course along the superior border of the pancreatic body (Fig. 4.8). In this way, the location and full extent of pancreatic pathology can be defined, and involvement of the peripancreatic structures determined. The retropancreatic area can be assessed for the presence of any enlarged lymph nodes.

Acute pancreatitis and its complications

As has been previously indicated (see Chapter 2), intraoperative ultrasonography may have a role in the detection of choledocholithiasis in the patient submitted to surgery for a complication of acute pancreatitis. Laparoscopic ultrasonography may be useful in the detection of common bile duct stones in the patient undergoing laparoscopic cholecystectomy for gallstone disease which is known to have given rise to acute pancreatitis (Fig. 4.9).

For the patient undergoing surgery for peripancreatic infection we have found intraoperative ultrasonography useful in assessing the pancreas and for accurately localising abscess, which require surgical drainage. Such collections are often loculated and ultrasound scanning will determine whether residual loculi require to be further explored.

Intraoperative ultrasonography is a useful investigative tool to have available when surgery is being undertaken to drain a pancreatic pseudocyst. The cyst can be scanned by placing the probe directly over it, but in the majority of cases the cyst will project into the posterior wall of the stomach, over which the transducer is positioned (Fig. 4.10(a)). The relationship of the cyst wall and the stomach can be ascertained and the location of the pancreatic vessels determined. In some instances, the examination may demonstrate that the cyst may be better drained by some other route. If, for example,

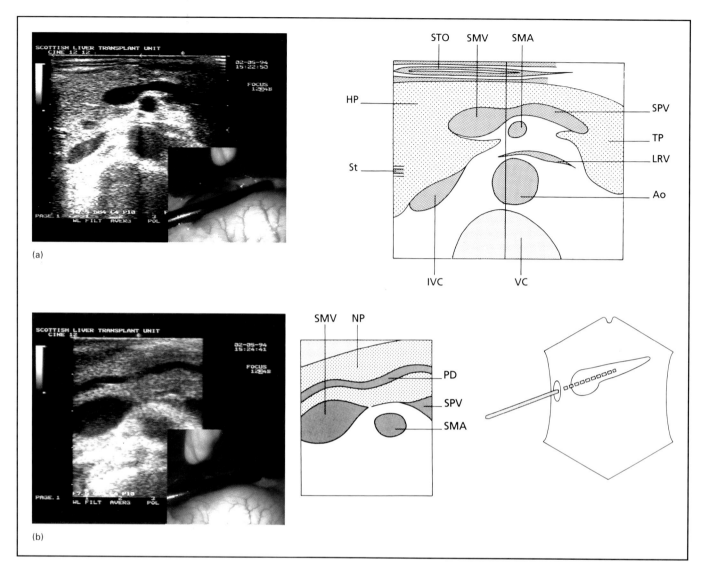

Fig. 4.8 Transverse/oblique laparoscopic sonograms orientated in the long axis of a normal pancreas in a patient presenting with hilar cholangiocarcinoma. (a) The relationships between the retropancreatic blood vessels and the head (HP), neck (NP) and body of the gland are demonstrated. A biliary stent (St) identifies the course of the common bile duct through the HP. (b) The pancreatic duct (PD) diameter is at the upper limit of normal (3 mm) and is demonstrated lengthwise traversing the NP. STO, stomach; SMV, superior mesenteric vein; SMA, superior mesenteric artery; SPV, splenic vein; TP, tail of pancreas; LRV, left renal vein; Ao, aorta; VC, vertebral column; IVC, inferior vena cava.

the cyst is more posteriorly placed, cystgastrostomy may not be safely undertaken and drainage into a Roux limb of jejunum may be preferable (Fig. 4.10(b)).

At the present time, laparoscopic intervention has not been considered for patients requiring pancreatic necrosectomy, but if this were to be undertaken the addition of ultrasound would be useful in planning the surgical

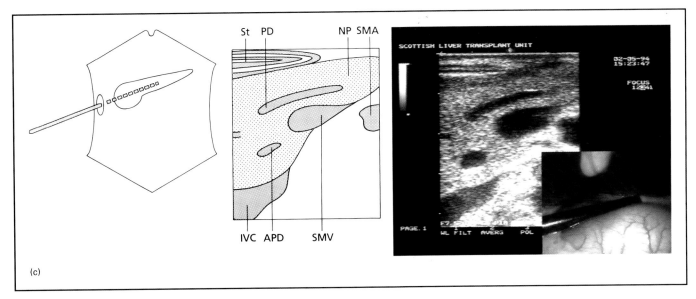

Fig. 4.8 (*Continued*) (c) The accessory pancreatic duct (APD) is identified passing superiorly from the uncinate process through the HP. Ao, aorta; IVC, inferior vena cava; LRV, left renal vein; SMA, superior mesenteric artery; SMV, superior mesenteric vein; SPV, splenic vein; STO, stomach; TP, tail of pancreas; VC, vertebral column.

approach. Similarly, laparoscopic approaches to pancreatic pseudocysts ought to be better directed by laparoscopic ultrasonography.

Chronic pancreatitis

In the operative management of chronic pancreatitis, intraoperative ultrasonography has been employed to help exclude the presence of coexisting pancreatic malignancy and is useful in planning the surgical approach. Pancreatic and bile duct dilatation may be defined with precision, thus guiding the surgeon in bypass procedures such as the pancreaticojejunostomy for intractable pancreatic pain (Fig. 4.11).

Fig. 4.9 Laparoscopic sonogram obtained during laparoscopic cholecystectomy in a patient whose previous attack of gallstone associated acute pancreatitis had been managed by endoscopic retrograde cholangiography and sphincterotomy. The scan is orientated in the long axis of the hepatic pedicle and demonstrates the common bile duct (CBD) containing one of several small calculi. CYD, cystic duct; PV, portal vein.

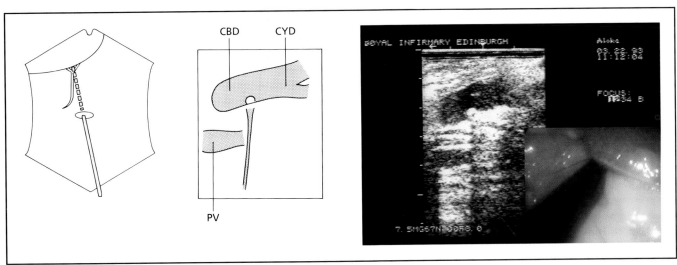

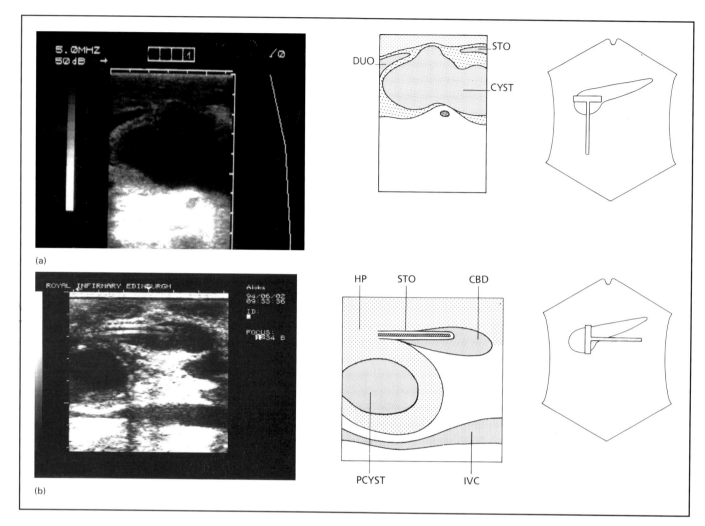

Fig. 4.10 (a) Transverse intraoperative sonogram obtained with the 5-MHz T-probe positioned on the stomach (STO) and first part of duodenum (DUO). The pseudocyst wall can be seen to lie directly behind the posterior wall of the STO. Note the projections of necrotic debris extending into the hypoechoic fluid within the cyst. (b) With the T-probe positioned along the free edge of the lesser omentum, a recurrent pancreatic pseudocyst (PCYST) has been demonstrated lying posteriorly within the pancreatic head (HP) and causing biliary obstruction. The common bile duct (CBD) has been decompressed by the insertion of a biliary endoprosthesis (ST). Downward pressure from the probe has caused indentation of the inferior vena cava (IVC).

Islet cell tumours

A number of workers [15–17] regard intraoperative ultrasound examination as the optimal method of locating neuroendocrine tumours of the pancreas, since these are not reliably localised by conventional radiological imaging. It is important to examine the entire gland since such lesions may be multifocal. Exposure of the gland may be undertaken by transection of the gastrocolic ligament and mobilisation of the colon at its splenic and hepatic flexures. Palpation of the head of the pancreas is facilitated by mobi-

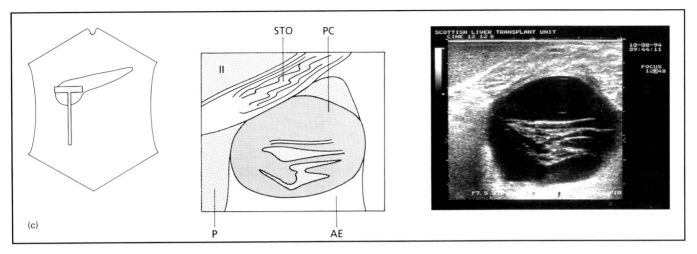

Fig. 4.10 (*Continued*) (c) Transverse intraoperative sonogram obtained with the probe placed upon the left hepatic lobe. A 6-cm diameter pseudocyst (PC) has been demonstrated arising from the pancreatic body (P) and indenting the posterior wall of the STO. Note the echogenic debris within the PC and the posterior acoustic enhancement (AE).

lising the duodenum at its lateral peritoneal attachment. These lesions usually appear as well-circumscribed hypoechoic lesions, but are occasionally hyperechoic (Fig. 4.12). Examination of the entire gland should be undertaken, sweeping the linear-array transducer along the length of the gland in both transverse and sagittal directions following careful mobilisation and palpation.

Although some experienced pancreatic surgeons may detect a number of these 'occult' insulinomas by palpation, the availability of state of the art high-resolution ultrasound systems has almost made redundant the use of extensive preoperative localisation studies [15–17]. Sensitivities for intraoperative ultrasound range from 83 to 100% compared with 42–88% for palpation alone [15]. None the less, it is likely that a combination of both careful palpation and a systematic intraoperative ultrasound examination is required to maximise the sensitivity of this approach. van Heerden *et al.* [16] reported that intraoperative ultrasonography detected insulinomas in nine of 13 patients with occult lesions, although the tumours were actually palpable in all but one of the patients.

In the era of minimal access surgery it was inevitable that the use of laparoscopy and laparoscopic ultrasonography would be considered in the detection of such tumours [12]. However, the rationale for the use of laparoscopic ultrasonography in the preoperative detection of pancreatic insulinoma is questionable if it is not envisaged that the lesion be removed by laparoscopic means. Conversely, staging laparoscopy with laparoscopic ultrasonography may be appropriate in the detection of intra-abdominal dissemination of a gastrinoma. We have already avoided an unnecessary laparotomy in one such patient who had been thought to have a large gastrinoma localised within the head of the pancreas.

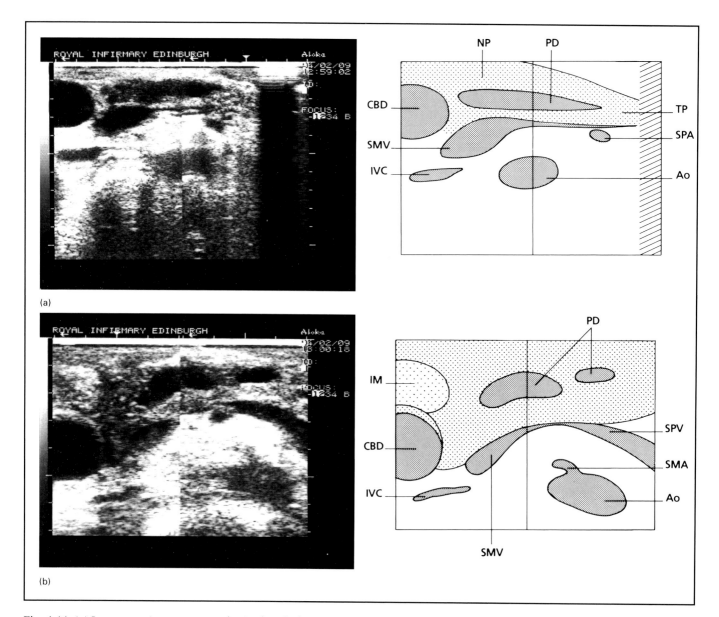

Fig. 4.11 (a) Intraoperative sonogram obtained with the 7.5-MHz T-probe placed transversely on the pancreas in a patient with both pancreatic duct and biliary obstruction secondary to chronic pancreatitis. The grossly dilated common bile duct (CBD) measuring approximately 30 mm in diameter is demonstrated in cross-section behind the pancreatic head. A distended and tortuous pancreatic duct (PD) is demonstrated extending to the atrophic body and tail (TP) of the gland, and this was opened longitudinally before fashioning a pancreaticojejunostomy. (b) A more caudal scan at the level of the origin of the superior mesenteric artery (SMA) from the aorta (Ao) identifies a hyperechoic chronic inflammatory mass (IM) within the pancreatic head as the cause of the ductal obstruction. IVC, inferior vena cava; NP, neck of pancreas; SMV, superior mesenteric vein; SPA, splenic artery; SPV, splenic vein. The probe position used in (a) and (b) is the same as that used for Fig. 4.12(a).

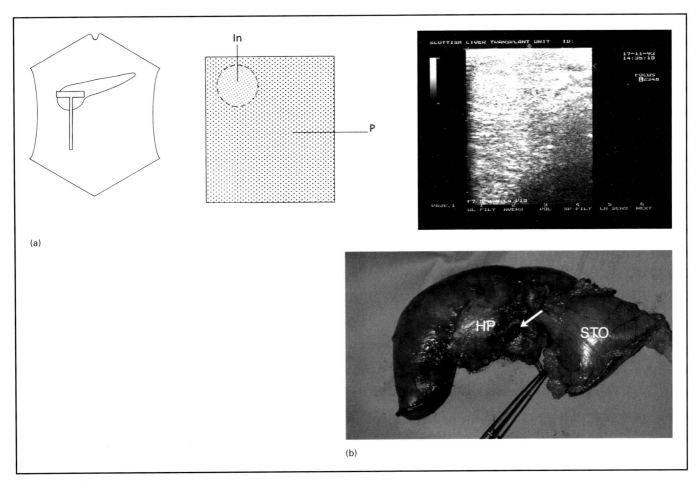

Fig. 4.12 (a) Intra-abdominal ultrasonography was undertaken with a 7.5-MHz linear-array transducer placed transversely on the body of the pancreas in a patient with intermittent episodes of hypoglycaemia, but in whom neither preoperative localisation studies nor operative palpation of the pancreas had identified the tumour site. A hyperechoic well-defined 10-mm diameter insulinoma (In) was identified within the pancreatic head (HP). (b) The decision was therefore made to perform pancreatico-duodenectomy whereby complete excision of the impalpable tumour was achieved (arrowed). P, pancreas; STO, stomach.

Pancreatic and periampullary cancer

The pancreas is a difficult organ to evaluate radiologically because of its retroperitoneal location. This gives rise to considerable difficulty in achieving accurate tumour staging preoperatively and in the selection of patients for exploratory laparotomy with a view to pancreatic resection with curative intent. Operative ultrasonography may be used to define the location and extent of the tumour and to evaluate its secondary effects on the biliary and pancreatic ducts and adjacent vasculature in patients submitted to open operation. However, the greater impact upon the management of patients with malignant biliary obstruction is now attributable to laparoscopic ultrasonography since this modality may avoid unnecessary laparotomy in a substantial proportion of patients with irresectable disease.

Intraoperative ultrasonography

At laparotomy, intraoperative ultrasound may be helpful in establishing the diagnosis in patients with obstructive jaundice where this has not been satisfactorily achieved preoperatively. Once the underlying lesion has been characterised, guided needle biopsy of the suspicious area may be undertaken, thereby increasing the safety of the procedure and improving the diagnostic

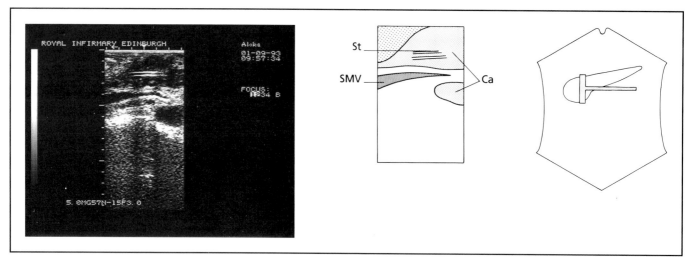

yield. Local invasion of the retroperitoneal tissues and adjacent organs can be defined, and identification of anatomical landmarks facilitates trial dissection of the tumour. The peripancreatic vasculature may be examined for evidence of occlusion, encasement or invasion which might render further exploration hazardous and fruitless. As described in Chapter 3, intraoperative ultrasound examination of the liver combined with direct palpation represents the most sensitive method for the detection of occult metastatic lesions, and this represents an important facet to the operative assessment of patients with malignant obstructive jaundice.

The finding of an obliterated terminal portion of both the common bile duct and pancreatic duct with proximal 'double-duct' dilatation is usually pathognomonic of pancreatic or periampullary carcinoma. The sonographic appearances of pancreatic carcinoma are typically those of a heterogeneous and hypoechoic mass which may cast dense acoustic shadows posteriorly (Figs 4.13 and 4.14). Hypoechoity is very suggestive of adenocarcinoma whereas hyperechoity may be caused by pancreatitis which is often present in the patient who has previously undergone diagnostic or therapeutic endoscopic retrograde cholangiopancreatography (ERCP). However, pancreatic and periampullary carcinomas may occasionally appear isoechoic (Fig. 4.15) or hyperechoic. Enlarged regional lymph nodes may be identified and sampled for frozen section histology.

Other workers have shown [4,13] that operative ultrasound examination is invaluable in assessing regional lymph node involvement, direct invasion of the adjacent tissues or invasion and encasement of the superior mesenteric and portal veins. Machi *et al.* [18] have reported that intraoperative ultrasound scanning is more specific (86 versus 56%) and accurate (90 versus 64%) than preoperative transabdominal ultrasound, dynamic CT scanning and angiography in assessing portal vein invasion in patients with carcinoma of the pancreatic head. None the less, the majority of surgeons currently seem unconvinced by these enthusiasts, and prefer to evaluate tumour resectability at open operation by mobilisation of the pancreas with trial dissection of the tumour.

Fig. 4.13 Intraoperative sonogram demonstrating a well-defined hypoechoic pancreatic carcinoma (Ca), within which a biliary stent (St) has been identified within the occluded common bile duct. In this sagittal cut angled across the pancreatic neck, the tumour is seen to be encasing the superior mesenteric vein (SMV), which becomes attenuated and stenosed with tumour invasion.

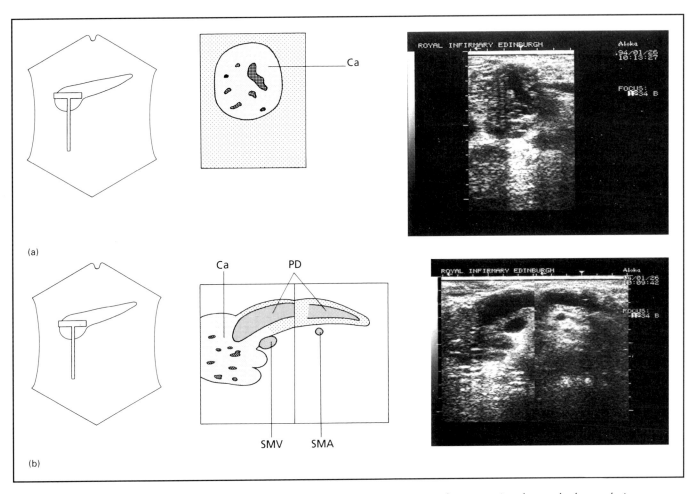

Fig. 4.14 (a) Intraoperative sonogram demonstrating the patchy hypoechoic appearance of a pancreatic carcinoma (Ca) measuring approximately 50 mm within the pancreatic head. (b) A transverse sonogram in the long axis of the pancreas in the same patient, demonstrates the tumour situated within the head of the gland causing obstruction of a dilated pancreatic duct (PD). The tumour is seen encroaching upon the superior mesenteric vein (SMV) posteriorly. SMA, superior mesenteric artery.

Laparoscopic ultrasonography

Several authors [6,7,19] have stressed the inability of conventional pre-operative techniques to detect occult metastatic deposits within the peritoneal cavity and liver. Discovery of such lesions at the time of laparotomy will curtail the intended operative procedure, whilst their non-detection before resectional surgery results in early tumour recurrence. Such limitations of existing non-invasive imaging techniques provide a strong rationale for recommending routine staging laparoscopy before consideration of operative intervention [7,19].

In the patient with suspected pancreatic malignancy the laparoscopic examination commences with a thorough inspection of the peritoneal surfaces, the capsule of the liver and the other viscera in order to identify the appear-

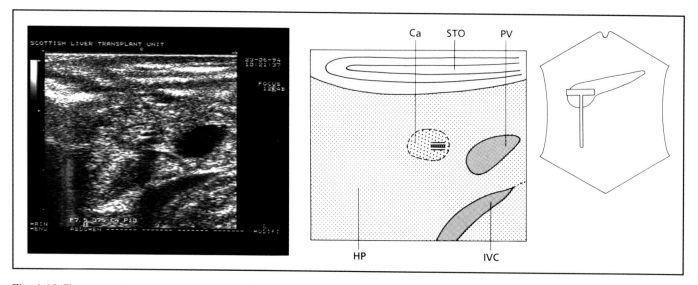

Fig. 4.15 Transverse intraoperative sonogram through the stomach (STO) and head of the pancreas (HP) demonstrating a small (less than 10 mm) isoechoic carcinoma (Ca) within which a biliary stent is identifiable. The portal vein (PV) and inferior vena cava (IVC) appear free from tumour invasion, and a pancreatoduodenectomy was successfully performed.

ances of peritoneal seedlings and obtain biopsy evidence of disseminated malignancy (Fig. 4.16). In the patient with locally advanced pancreatic carcinoma, there may be invasion of the portal, superior mesenteric or splenic veins. The laparoscopic appearances of dilated splanchnic veins should therefore raise suspicion as to the presence of segmental portal hypertension secondary to local tumour invasion (Fig. 4.17). It is useful to use the laparoscopic ultrasound transducer as a palpating probe to identify any retrogastric mass lesions, and to elevate the left hepatic lobe in order to inspect its undersurface, the caudate lobe of the liver and the lesser omentum

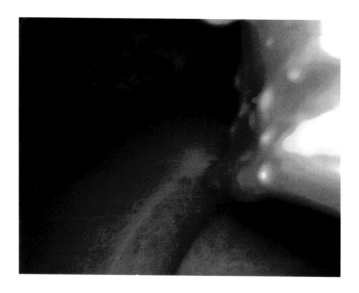

Fig. 4.16 Staging laparoscopy in a patient considered on the basis of preoperative transabdominal ultrasound and CT scans to have a resectable tumour in the head of the pancreas. Note the numerous small metastatic deposits on the surface of the falciform ligament and diaphragmatic peritoneum.

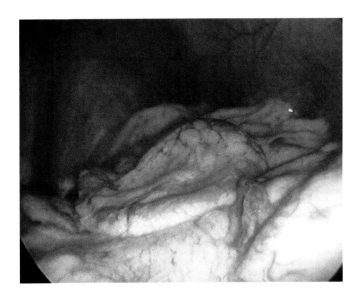

Fig. 4.17 Laparoscopic examination of the peritoneal cavity in a patient with tumour invasion of the portal vein. Note the dilated tortuous venous collaterals.

for lymphadenopathy. However, we do not routinely enter the lesser sac to evaluate resectability of lesions in the pancreatic head and prefer to minimise displacement of the viscera at the outset of the examination to avoid gaseous attenuation of the ultrasound scans. As with the intra-abdominal staging assessment of any malignant process, a careful examination of the liver is performed at the outset to confirm or exclude metastatic disease. The high-resolution images of laparoscopic ultrasonography make easy the diagnosis of intrahepatic duct dilatation, and provide a very sensitive means of detecting intrahepatic tumour deposits (Fig. 4.18). Nevertheless, it should

Fig. 4.18 Staging laparoscopic ultrasound examination in a patient thought on the basis of dynamic spiral CT scanning to have a potentially resectable carcinoma of the pancreatic head. A 14-mm diameter intrahepatic metastasis (MET) in segment IV and displaying the typical 'bull's-eye' appearance was discovered. This lesion was not apparent on laparoscopic inspection of the liver. RPV, right portal vein.

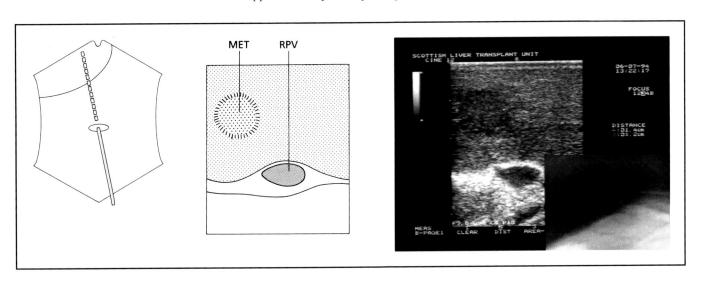

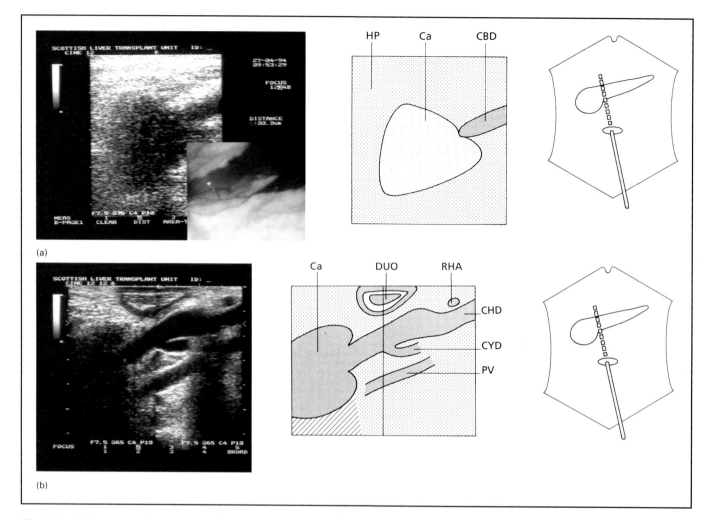

Fig. 4.19 (a) Laparoscopic sonograms demonstrating a hypoechoic carcinoma (Ca) within the head of the pancreas (HP), measuring 30 mm and causing obstruction of the common bile duct (CBD). (b) A composite sagittally orientated scan demonstrates the passage of the dilated duct and portal vein (PV) behind the first part of the duodenum (DUO) to the level of the tumour in the HP. Note that the confluence of the cystic duct (CYD) and common hepatic duct (CHD) is free from tumour infiltration. RHA, right hepatic artery.

be recognised that pneumobilia following previous biliary stenting or sphincterotomy may cause acoustic interference and so degrade the images.

Laparoscopy is very limited in its ability to provide precise information regarding the status of tumour invasion into retroperitoneal structures unless the tumour is very obviously advanced, and direct visualisation of small tumours of the pancreatic head or periampullary region is virtually impossible. This may normally be achieved at an early stage in the laparoscopic ultrasound examination with the probe inserted in the umbilical port, and the transducer positioned upon the pancreatic head and guided by the laparoscope via the right lateral port. As described earlier, pancreatic carcinomas

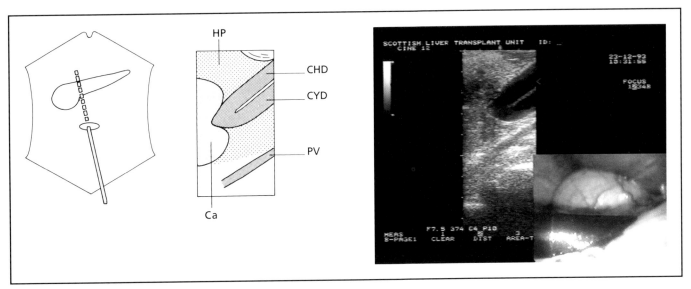

Fig. 4.20 Sagittal laparoscopic sonogram demonstrating a 40-mm carcinoma (Ca) of the pancreatic head (HP) causing biliary obstruction immediately distal to the confluence of cystic (CYD) and common hepatic ducts (CHD). This patient would not, therefore, be suitable for a palliative biliary bypass utilising the gallbladder as a conduit. PV, portal vein.

are usually densely hypoechoic and well circumscribed (Fig. 4.19) compared with the surrounding pancreatic parenchyma which has a similar echo texture to that of the liver. The tumour can be located by following the dilated or stented common bile duct inferiorly into the pancreas from the porta hepatis (Figs 4.19(b) and 4.20), and using the adjacent portal vein as a useful reference landmark for the neck of the gland.

The presence of a periampullary carcinoma may be inferred from the presence of dilatation of both the common bile duct and pancreatic ducts without neccessarily obtaining images of a space occupying lesion within the pancreas (Fig. 4.21). Periampullary lesions may be difficult to define because of their projection into the lumen of the second part of the duodenum. However, if care is taken to avoid acoustic interference associated with intraduodenal gas, debris and peristaltic movements, it is usually possible to define the primary lesion (Fig. 4.22). Conversely, the absence of pancreatic duct dilatation in the patient with malignant obstruction of the intrapancreatic portion of the common bile duct strongly suggests a diagnosis of cholangiocarcinoma. Care must be exercised in the diagnosis of cystic pancreatic lesions as cystic carcinomas can occasionally masquerade as benign postinflammatory lesions and a tissue diagnosis should be obtained whenever doubt exists (Fig. 4.23).

Direct extrapancreatic invasion of tumour into the retroperitoneum, root of the mesentery or adjacent viscera should be evaluated. Well-circumscribed tumours may be defined extending outwith the limits of the pancreas (Fig. 4.24). However, local tumour advancement is more commonly inferred by

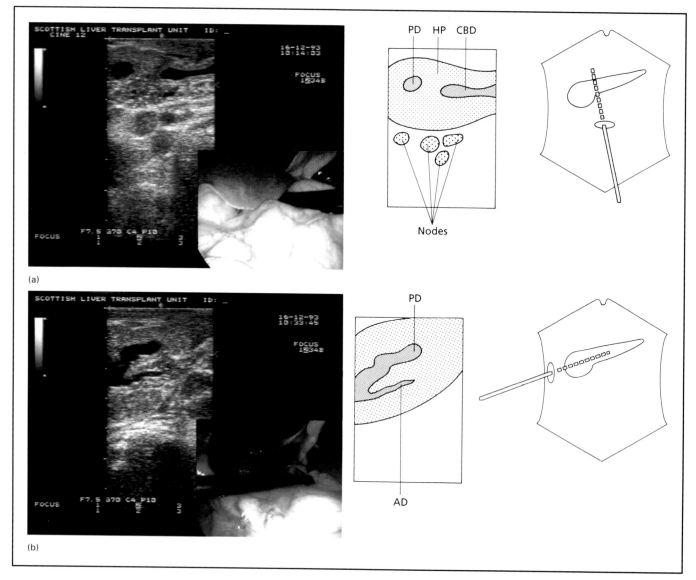

Fig. 4.21 (a) Sagittal section through the pancreatic head (HP) in a patient presenting with a periampullary carcinoma. Note the dilated pancreatic duct (PD) and common bile duct (CBD), and a cluster of enlarged lymph nodes in the retropancreatic region. (b) A transverse laparoscopic sonogram obtained with the probe inserted through the right lateral port in the same patient demonstrates the confluence of the dilated pancreatic and accessory pancreatic ducts (AD) within the HP.

the demonstration of an extensive tumour mass measuring greater than 5 cm in maximum diameter and associated with indistinct margins indicative of malignant infiltration.

For the pancreaticobiliary surgeon, portal vein patency is of great significance and assessment of the peripancreatic vasculature is, therefore, an important component of staging laparoscopic ultrasonography in determining the resectability of carcinomas of the pancreatic head and periampullary region. The portal, splenic and superior mesenteric veins and the hepatic and superior mesenteric arteries should all be carefully examined for

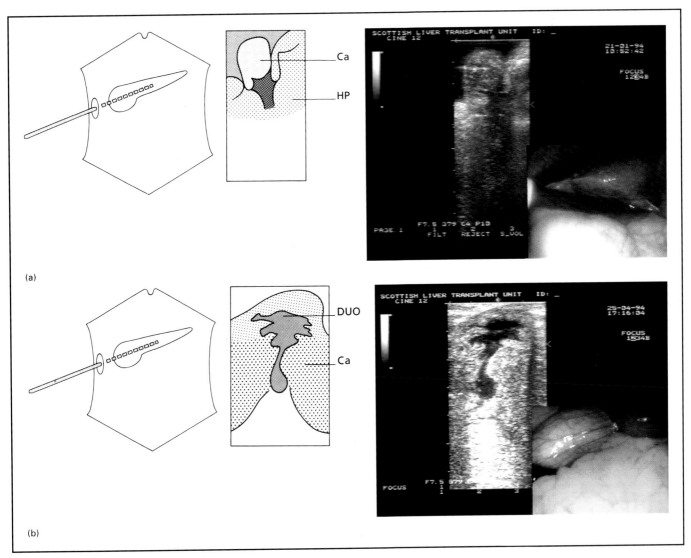

Fig. 4.22 (a) With the laparoscopic ultrasound transducer placed gently upon the duodenum, a 20-mm diameter periampullary carcinoma (Ca) is demonstrated prolapsing into the duodenal (DUO) lumen. (b) Some periampullary tumours are large and sessile and can be seen invading the pancreatic parenchyma. HP, head of the pancreas.

evidence of tumour invasion. Criteria employed in determining vascular invasion during high-resolution contact ultrasonography are: (i) vascular occlusion with failure to demonstrate a patent vessel; (ii) a fixed stenosis of the vessel indicating tumour encasement; and (iii) direct invasion of the vessel wall indicated by loss of the hyperechoic tissue interface between tumour and the adventitia of the artery or vein, or the demonstration of tumour encroaching upon the vessel lumen. The relationships between the pancreatic tumour and the vessels passing between the porta hepatis, neck of pancreas and root of mesentery should be examined in both sagittal and transverse planes (Figs 4.25–4.27). Care must be taken not to apply excessive down

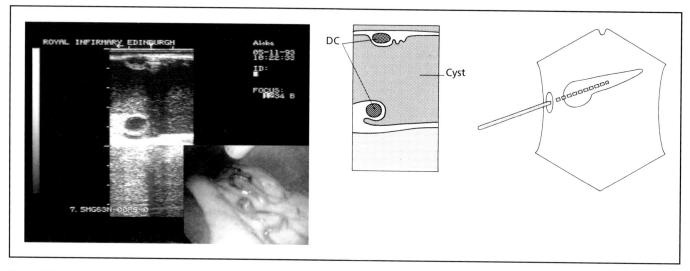

Fig. 4.23 Laparoscopic sonogram orientated along the length of the pancreas demonstrating a large cystic lesion within the pancreatic body. The presence of daughter cysts (DC) within the cyst wall characterises it as an adenocystic carcinoma of the pancreas, later confirmed by biopsy.

pressure with the ultrasound probe since the major venous structures are normally easily compressible and the impression of tumour stenosis may be erroneously created. If difficulty is encountered in maintaining satisfactory transducer contact without undue compression of the underlying tissues, the instillation of warm crystalloid solution into the peritoneal cavity can be used to optimise acoustic coupling.

Fig. 4.24 Sagittal laparoscopic sonogram through the neck of the pancreas (NP) demonstrating a carcinoma (Ca) arising from the head of the pancreas and extending cephalad into tissues of the hepatoduodenal ligament. Although extending close alongside the portal vein (PV), no direct tumour invasion was evident. The findings of irresectability due to extrapancreatic tumour invasion were later confirmed at laparotomy. Hepatic segment I (caudate lobe); St, biliary stent.

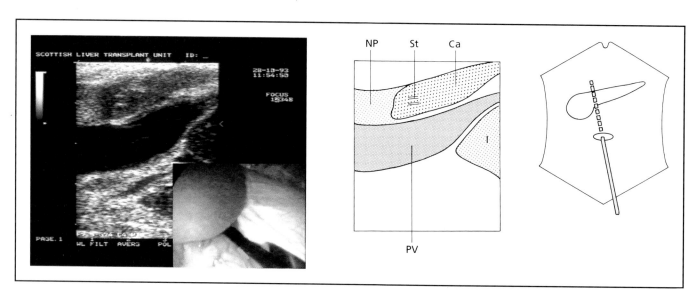

Fig. 4.25 Sagittal laparoscopic sonogram through the first part of the duodenum (D_1) and neck of the pancreas (NP) with the probe inserted through the umbilical port. Tumour (Ca) can be seen extending posteriorly into the uncinate process (UP) and close to the superior mesenteric vein (SMV). However, the vein–tumour interface is preserved and no direct vascular invasion can be inferred from this image. PD, pancreatic duct.

Colour flow Doppler ultrasound is an option which may facilitate the recognition of and demonstrate patency within the peripancreatic blood vessels (Fig. 4.28).

Occlusion of the portal venous inflow to the liver frequently results in cavernous transformation within the porta hepatis, recognised as multiple interconnecting venous channels in the absence of a recognisable patient main portal vein (Fig. 4.29).

The porta hepatis and para-aortic regions should be assessed for lymphadenopathy. It is our own preference to undertake this part of the examination with the laparoscopic probe in the umbilical port (Fig. 4.30). As with other staging investigations, the sonographic appearances of lymph node enlargement alone are not specific enough to diagnose malignant invasion, given that lymphadenopathy is frequently observed secondary to the inflammatory reaction associated with pancreatic carcinoma, or as a consequence of endoscopic stenting. Accessible lymph nodes can be sampled by fine needle aspiration under laparoscopic ultrasound guidance for cytological examination (Fig. 4.31).

Our own experience with staging laparoscopic ultrasonography in the assessment of patients with pancreatic or periampullary carcinoma now extends to some 60 patients to date. In an early report [10], staging laparoscopy was performed in a cohort of 40 consecutive patients with pancreatic or periampullary carcinoma who were considered, on the basis of preceding transabdominal ultrasound or CT scans, to be potentially suitable candidates for pancreatic resection. Occult metastatic lesions were demonstrated in 14 patients (35%) by laparoscopy alone (Table 4.1).

Laparoscopic ultrasonography was also performed in 38 patients. Satisfactory images of the primary tumour were obtained in 31 patients (81%). In 23 patients (59%), laparoscopic ultrasonography demonstrated factors which confirmed the irresectable nature of the tumour (Table 4.2).

In this same group of 38 patients, staging information in addition to that provided by laparoscopy alone was obtained in 20 patients (53%), changing

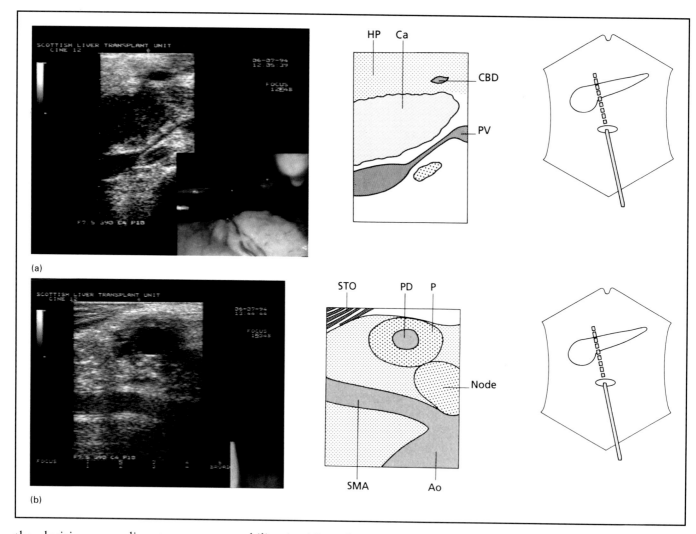

the decision regarding tumour resectability in 10 patients (25%). The combination of laparoscopy and laparoscopic ultrasonography was more specific and accurate than versus laparoscopy alone in predicting tumour resectability. The impact of staging laparoscopy with laparoscopic ultrasonography in the management of this series of patients with 'potentially resectable' disease is illustrated in Fig. 4.32. Twenty-two patients underwent laparotomy with an overall resectability rate of 30% in this highly selected group. However, it should be recognised that laparotomy was performed in many of these patients, despite the laparoscopic ultrasound findings, in order to validate the accuracy of this novel diagnostic modality (Fig. 4.32). The 'unnecessary laparotomy' rate might be expected to diminish as staging laparoscopic ultrasonography becomes accepted within rationalised staging algorithms.

Of those investigations traditionally employed in the selection of patients with pancreatic and periampullary carcinoma for resectional surgery, ultrasonography is non-invasive but highly operator dependent. It can confirm the presence of extrahepatic biliary obstruction and will screen the liver for metastatic disease. It can be at least as accurate as CT scanning in determining local resectability of pancreatic cancer [20,21]. However, these

Fig. 4.26 (a) A narrow fixed stenosis of the portal vein (PV) due to malignant encasement by a carcinoma (Ca) of the pancreatic head (HP) is demonstrated. (b) Displacement of the probe leftwards over the neck of the gland demonstrates the superior mesenteric artery (SMA), which appears patent and uninvolved by tumour, although a nodal mass is apparent adjacent to its origin from the aorta (Ao). Note the dilated pancreatic duct (PD) within an atrophic distal pancreas (P). CBD, common bile duct; STO, stomach.

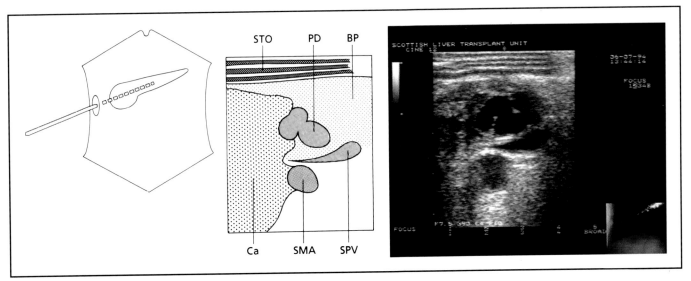

Fig. 4.27 Transverse laparoscopic sonogram demonstrating occlusion of a dilated pancreatic duct (PD) at the level of the pancreatic neck by a large tumour (Ca). Tumour invasion of the superior mesenteric artery (SMA) and splenic vein (SPV) is demonstrated in this scan. BP, body of pancreas; STO, stomach.

results have not been widely reproduced, and in practice inadequate imaging of the retroperitoneal structures is a frequent occurrence [22]. CT has been shown by some to be too inaccurate to recommend its use alone as a staging investigation [23,24], although it also is operator dependent in the interpretation of the images, which in turn depend on the method of administration of contrast enhancement and the speed of image acquisition. Selective visceral angiography has been reported as both an accurate means of defining irresectability and potentially misleading in predicting tumour resectability [25,26]. In the present study we used angiography primarily as a means of validating the findings of laparoscopic ultrasonography regarding vascular invasion.

Use of laparoscopic ultrasonography to assess pancreatic malignancy seems logical. The detailed view of the peritoneal cavity at laparoscopy is superior to that provided by any other contemporary investigation in detecting tiny peritoneal tumour deposits and liver metastases [24,27], but the laparoscopist is limited in his/her ability to assess the primary tumour and its locoregional stage. Although direct laparoscopic inspection of pancreatic tumours from within the lesser sac has been well described by both infragastric [28,29] and supragastric routes [30–32] and whilst recognising that this may be useful in the diagnosis and biopsy of tumours of the body and tail of the pancreas, it is not in practice a suitable means of assessing resectability of small inaccessible tumours within the head of the gland. However, we found that laparoscopic ultrasonography consistently provided highly detailed images of the pancreas and neighbouring retroperitoneal structures. Accordingly, it was possible to demonstrate the signs of local tumour invasion, peripancreatic lymphadenopathy and vascular invasion.

Several authors have also reported the use of laparoscopic ultrasonography to confirm the presence of primary pancreatic tumours and accurately define hepatobiliary and pancreatic anatomy [33–35]. Endosonography relies upon similar principles to laparoscopic ultrasonography, whereby high-resolution ultrasound transducers are introduced into direct apposition with

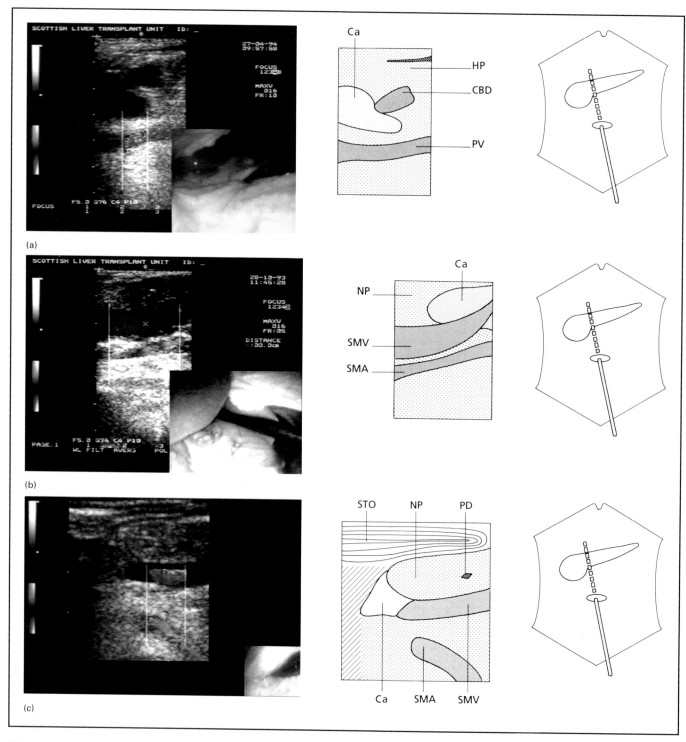

Fig. 4.28 (a) Colour flow laparoscopic ultrasound demonstrating the passage of the portal vein (PV) near a carcinoma (Ca) of the pancreatic head (HP). (b) The opposing directions of the blood flow within the superior mesenteric artery (SMA) and vein (SMV) behind the neck of the pancreas (NP) are demonstrated in red and blue. (c) A fixed stenosis of the SMV due to Ca encasement has been demonstrated. Occlusion of the SMV by direct Ca invasion from the uncinate process is demonstrated in this colour-enhanced laparoscopic sonogram. CBD, common bile duct; PD, pancreatic duct; STO, stomach.

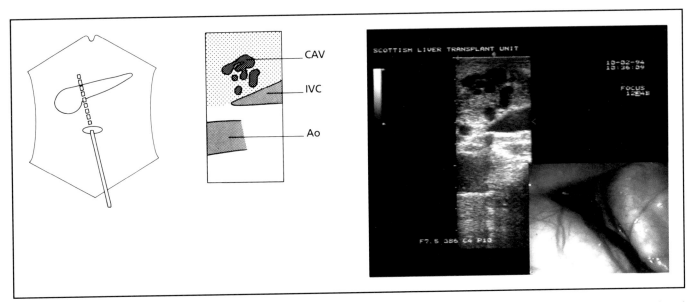

Fig. 4.29 Cavernous transformation (CAV) of the portal vein in a patient with a locally advanced pancreatic carcinoma. Ao, aorta; IVC, inferior vena cava.

the tissues under investigation, in this case via the stomach and duodenal wall. Impressive results have been reported in the assessment of tumour size, lymph node status and vascular invasion in patients with pancreatic and periampullary carcinomas [36,37]. However, endosonography cannot be expected to detect peritoneal and liver metastases, and this is reflected in its overall accuracy of 66% in the tumour node metastasis staging of pancreatic cancer [37]. This inability to define malignant dissemination within the peritoneal cavity must limit the usefulness of endosonography alongside laparoscopic ultrasonography within the algorithm of investigations. We

Fig. 4.30 Sagittal laparoscopic sonogram obtained with the probe inserted through the umbilical port and transducer placed upon the first part of the duodenum (D_1). The portal vein (PV) and superior mesenteric artery (SMA) are demonstrated in their passage behind the neck of the pancreas (NP) which appears atrophic with a dilated pancreatic duct (PD). Several enlarged lymph nodes were identified surrounding the PV in the hilar region, and confirmed to contain metastatic tumour at laparotomy.

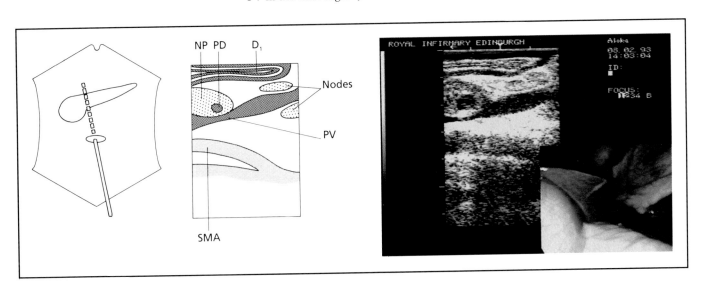

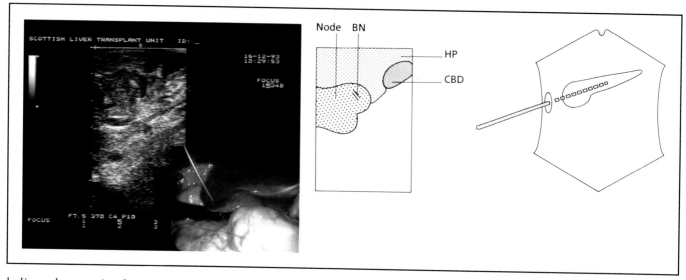

believe that staging laparoscopy is indispensable in the preoperative assessment of such patients, and that laparoscopic ultrasonography presents the means whereby the number of preoperative investigations may be rationalised and surgical intervention better tailored to the patients needs.

Fig. 4.31 Laparoscopic ultrasound guided fine needle aspiration of a 20-mm lymph node mass behind the pancreatic head (HP). The needle point (BN) appears as a hyperechoic moving point in its passage through the tissues. CBD, common bile duct.

References

1 Carter DC. Cancer of the pancreas. *Gut* 1990; 31: 494–6.
2 Sigel B, Machi J, Anderson KW III, *et al.* Operative sonography of the biliary tree and pancreas. *Sem Ultrasound CT MR* 1985; 6: 2–14.
3 Klotter HJ, Rückert K, Kümmerle F, Rothmund M. The use of intraoperative sonography in endocrine tumours of the pancreas. *World J Surg* 1987; 11: 635–41.
4 Plainfosse MC, Bouillot JL, Rivaton F, Vaucamps P, Hernigou A, Alexandre JH. The use of operative sonography in carcinoma of the pancreas. *World J Surg* 1987; 11: 654–8.
5 Hernigou A, Plainfosse MC, Chapuis Y, *et al.* Operative ultrasound of the pancreas: a review of 53 cases. *J Belge Radiol* 1986; 69: 37–42.
6 Cuschieri A. Laparoscopy in diagnosis and staging of patients with cancer of the exocrine pancreas. In: Preece PE, Cuschieri A, Rosin RD, eds. *Cancer of the Bile Ducts and Pancreas*. Philadelphia: WB Saunders, 1989: 189–96.
7 Warshaw AL, Tepper JE, Shipley WU. Laparoscopy in the staging and planning of therapy for pancreatic cancer. *Am J Surg* 1986; 151: 76–80.

Outcome	Laparoscopy	
	Resectable	Irresectable
Resectable	12	0
Irresectable	14	14

Table 4.1 Prediction of resectability by staging laparoscopy in 40 patients with pancreatic or periampullary carcinoma. (After John *et al.* [10])

Sensitivity = 12/12 (100%). Specificity = 14/28 (50%). Accuracy = 26/40 (65%).

Table 4.2 Prediction of resectability by staging laparoscopy and laparoscopic ultrasonography in 38 patients with pancreatic or periampullary carcinoma. (After John *et al.* [10])

	Laparoscopy/laparoscopic sonography	
Outcome	Resectable	Irresectable
Resectable	11	1
Irresectable	3	23

Sensitivity = 11/12 (92%). Specificity = 23/26 (88%). Accuracy = 34/38 (89%).

8 John TG, Garden OJ. Assessment of pancreatic cancer. In: Cuesta M, Nagy AG, eds. *Minimally Invasive Surgery in Gastrointestinal Cancer.* London: Churchill Livingstone, 1993: 95–111.

9 John TG, Garden OJ. Laparoscopic ultrasound: extending the scope of diagnostic laparoscopy. *Br J Surg* 1994; 81: 5–6.

10 John TG, Greig JD, Carter DC, Garden OJ. Carcinoma of the pancreatic head and periampullary region: tumor staging with laparoscopy and laparoscopic ultrasonography. *Ann Surg* 1995; 2 (in press).

11 John TG, Garden OJ. Laparoscopic ultrasonography for staging of abdominal malignancy. In: Garden OJ, Paterson-Brown S, eds. *Principles and Practice of Surgical Laparoscopy.* London: WB Saunders, 1994: 565–83.

12 Pietrabissa A, Shimi SM, Vander Velpen G, Cuschieri A. Localisation of insulinoma by laparoscopic infragastric inspection of the pancreas and contact ultrasonography. *Surg Oncol* 1993; 2: 83–6.

13 Serio G, Fugazzola C, Iacono C, *et al.* Intraoperative ultrasonography in pancreatic cancer. *Int J Pancreatol* 1992; 11: 31–41.

14 Sigel B, Coelho JCU, Spigos D, Donahue PE, Wood DK, Nyhus L. Ultrasonic imaging during biliary and pancreatic surgery. *Am J Surg* 1981; 141: 84–9.

15 Zeiger MA, Shawker TH, Norton JA. Use of intraoperative ultrasonography to localize islet cell tumors. *World J Surg* 1993; 17: 448–54.

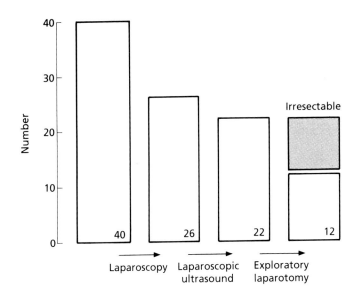

Fig. 4.32 Diagrammatic representation of the selection of patients for exploratory laparotomy and resection of carcinomas of the pancreatic head or periampullary region following staging laparoscopy and laparoscopic ultrasonography.

16 van Heerden JA, Grant CS, Czako PF, Service FJ, Charboneau JW. Occult functioning insulinomas: which localizing studies are indirected? *Surgery* 1992; 112: 1010–15.

17 Rothmund M. Localization of endocrine pancreatic tumours. *Br J Surg* 1994; 81: 164–6.

18 Machi J, Sigel B, Zaren HA, Kurohiji T, Yamashita Y. Operative ultrasonography during hepatobiliary and pancreatic surgery. *World J Surg* 1993; 17: 64–6.

19 Cuschieri A. Laparoscopy for pancreatic cancer: does it benefit the patient? *Eur J Surg Oncol* 1988; 14: 41–4.

20 Campbell JP, Wilson SR. Pancreatic neoplasms: how useful is evaluation with ultrasound. *Radiology* 1988; 167: 341–4.

21 Päivansalo M, Lähde S. Ultrasonography and CT in pancreatic malignancy. *Acta Radiol (Diagn)* 1988; 29: 343–4.

22 Shmulewitz A, Teefey SA, Robinson BS. Factors affecting image quality and diagnostic efficacy in abdominal sonography: a prospective study of 140 patients. *JCU* 1993; 21: 623–30.

23 Ross CB, Sharp KW, Kaufman AJ, Andrews T, Williams LF. Efficacy of computerised tomography in the preoperative staging of pancreatic carcinoma. *Am J Surg* 1988; 54: 221–6.

24 Bryde Anderson H, Effersoe H, Tjalve E, Burcharth F. CT for assessment of pancreatic and periampullary cancer. *Acta Radiol* 1993; 34: 569–72.

25 Appleton GVN, Cooper MJ, Bathurst NCG, Williamson RCN, Virjee J. The value of angiography in the surgical management of pancreatic disease. *Ann Roy Col Surg Engl* 1989; 71: 92–6.

26 Trede M, Schwall G, Saeger HD. Survival after pancreatoduodenectomy. 118 consecutive resections without an operative mortality. *Ann Surg* 1990; 211: 447–58.

27 Murugiah M, Windsor JA, Redhead D, *et al.* The role of selective visceral angiography in the management of pancreatic and periampullary cancer. *World J Surg* 1993; 17: 796–800.

28 Cuschieri A, Hall AW, Clark J. Value of laparoscopy in the diagnosis and management of pancreatic carcinoma. *Gut* 1978; 19: 672–7.

29 Strauch M, Lux G, Ottenjann R. Infragastric pancreoscopy. *Endoscopy* 1973; 5: 30–2.

30 Watanabe M, Takatori Y, Ueki K, *et al.* Pancreatic biopsy under visual control in conjunction with laparoscopy for diagnosis of pancreatic cancer. *Endoscopy* 1989; 21: 105–7.

31 Meyer-Berg J, Ziegler U, Kirstaedter HJ, Palme G. Peritoneoscopy in carcinoma of the pancreas. Report of 20 cases. *Endoscopy* 1973; 5: 86–90.

32 Ishida H, Dohzono T, Furukawa Y, Kobayashi M, Tsuneoka K. Laparoscopy and biopsy in the diagnosis of malignant intra-abdominal tumors. *Endoscopy* 1984; 16: 140–2.

33 Cuesta MA, Meijer S, Borgstein PJ, Sibinga Mulder L, Sikkenk AC. Laparoscopic ultrasonography for hepatobiliary and pancreatic malignancy. *Br J Surg* 1993; 80: 1571–4.

34 Jakimowicz JJ. Intraoperative ultrasonography during minimal access surgery. *J Roy Col Surg Edin* 1993; 38: 231–8.

35 Okita K, Kodama T, Oda M, Takemoto T. Laparoscopic ultrasonography. Diagnosis of liver and pancreatic cancer. *Scand J Gastroenterol* 1984; 19 (suppl. 94): 91–100.

36 Rösch T, Braig C, Gain T, *et al.* Staging of pancreatic and ampullary carcinoma by endoscopic ultrasonography. Comparison with conventional sonography, computed tomography, and angiography. *Gastroenterology* 1992; 102: 188–99.

37 Tio TL, Tytgat GNJ, Cikot RJLM, Houthoff HJ, Sars PRA. Ampullopancreatic carcinoma: preoperative TNM classification with endosonography. *Radiology* 1990; 175: 455–61.

5: Intraoperative and Laparoscopic Ultrasound: the Future

Although the concept of intraoperative contact sonography has been recognised since the 1960s, and has since become regarded by many hepatobiliary and pancreatic specialists as an indispensible operative tool, it has not been universally adopted with great enthusiasm by surgeons in general. The reasons for this include the relatively slow development of dedicated B-mode intraoperative ultrasound systems with high-resolution ultracompact probes which meet today's standards. There has also been an unwillingness by some surgeons to acquire skills in this unfamiliar technology, or to be seen to be transgressing on to the territory of the radiologist. However, the experience of surgeons working in a variety of specialities has shown that these problems can be overcome, so the future should witness increasing acceptance of invasive ultrasonography within the armamentarium of the general surgeon.

Ultrasound equipment

It has taken a considerable time for the manufacturers of ultrasound equipment to develop systems which are easily used in the operating theatre and provide images immediately acceptable to the operating surgeon. Although the option of using high-resolution ultrasound transducers intraoperatively has been available for many years, the large and cumbersome ultrasound machines to which the probes were connected were often a disadvantage in the operating theatre, and the seemingly complex instrumentation was often intimidating to the untrained assistant or circulating nurse. The capital outlay for such equipment often entailed that it be shared amongst a number of interested clinicians. Whereas the use of such machines by both surgeon and radiologist may be more cost efficient, the development of smaller and relatively inexpensive machines specifically for operative use was inevitable. Such portable equipment is currently available, but can also accommodate a variety of transabdominal and intraoperative ultrasound transducers.

Duplex sonography (i.e. ultrasound scanning which utilises Doppler waveform analysis simultaneously with real-time B-mode imaging) and colour Doppler scanning techniques have added a new dimension to ultrasonography in recent years. Although these techniques have found limited application other than in the field of vascular surgery, their use in other areas, such as in imaging the hepatic parenchyma and vasculature, is increasingly being recognised [1]. Inevitably, intraoperative and laparoscopic ultrasound probes have become available which incorporate this technology. The ability to rapidly 'sample' a structure and characterise the nature of its blood flow (e.g. as arterial, inferior vena caval or portal venous flow, or the absence of blood flow in the case of ductal structures) undoubtedly facilitates the rapid recognition of the intra-abdominal vasculature [2] (Figs 5.1 and 5.2), and

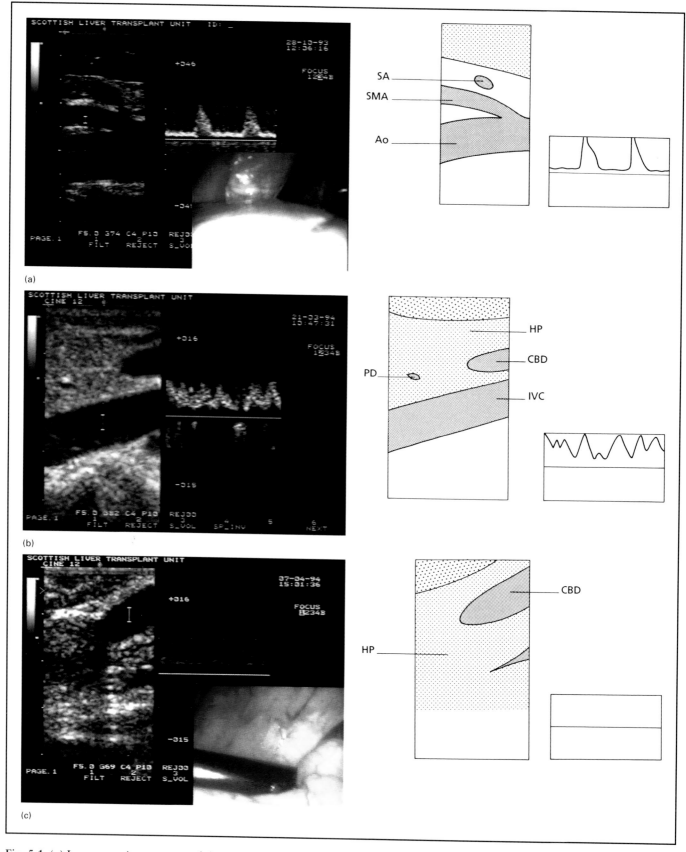

Fig. 5.1 (a) Laparoscopic sonogram of the para-aortic region obtained with the probe positioned upon the left hepatic lobe. The Doppler sampling 'gate' has been placed over the superior mesenteric artery (SMA) giving a typical arterial Doppler spectral waveform. (b) With the probe placed over the pancreatic head (HP), the characteristic Doppler waveform of the inferior vena cava (IVC) is seen representing venous pulsation transmitted from the right heart. (c) No detectable blood flow is present when the gate is positioned over the common bile duct (CBD). Ao, aorta; PD, pancreatic duct; SA, splenic artery. The probe position used in (a) is the same as that used in Fig. 4.18. The probe position used in (b) and (c) is the same as that used in Fig. 5.2(a).

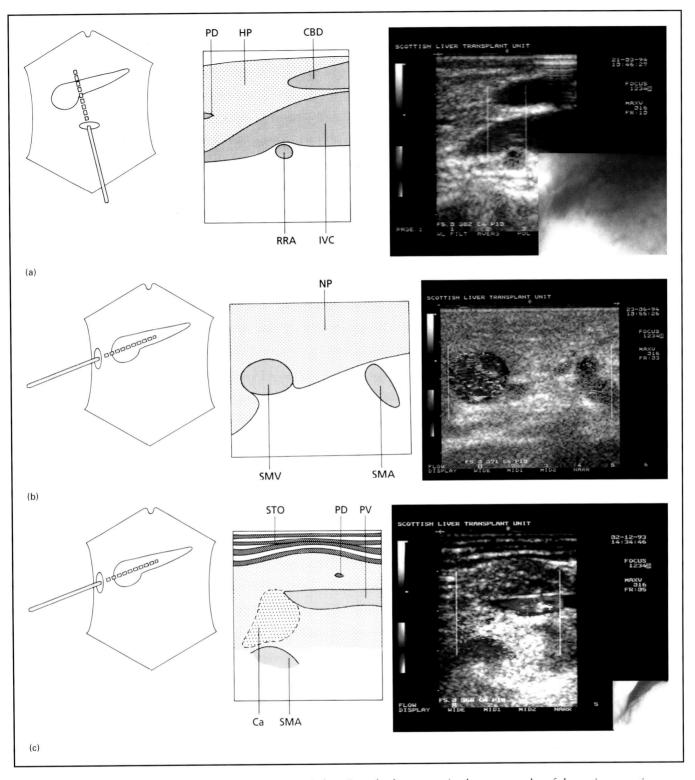

Fig. 5.2 (a) Colour Doppler laparoscopic ultrasonography of the peripancreatic vasculature. Blood flow within the inferior vena cava (IVC) and right renal artery (RRA) is demonstrated in red and blue, respectively. However, no colour enhancement occurs over the common bile duct (CBD) (cf. Fig. 4.6(a), Chapter 4). (b) A transverse scan in the long axis of the pancreas identifies the superior mesenteric vein (SMV) and artery (SMA) in colour passing behind the pancreatic neck (NP). Sagittal laparoscopic sonogram through the NP demonstrating the course of the portal vein (PV) and SMA in colour. (c) Venous invasion by a carcinoma (Ca) extending from the uncinate process of the pancreas is demonstrated by the stenotic segment of vein which does not enhance with colour. HP, head of the pancreas; PD, pancreatic duct; STO, stomach.

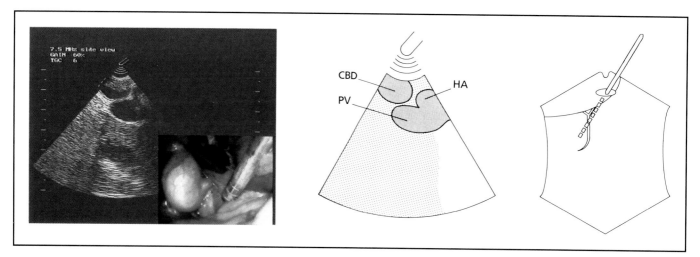

may aid in the assessment of vascular invasion in patients with intra-abdominal malignancy (Fig. 5.2(c)). However, such an advance does require a significant financial investment in equipment and may increase the complexity and duration of the examination.

Considerable advances have been made in the design of intraoperative transducers. Although there has been some debate amongst surgeons as to the relative advantages and disadvantages of linear-array and sectoral ultrasound transducers at open surgery, laparoscopic transducers are at an early stage of development having generally been adapted from existing intraoperative probes. It has yet to be established whether a universal laparoscopic transducer is feasible. Our own experience would suggest that a linear-array transducer configuration is necessary for examination of the liver, but convex curvilinear-array or sectoral transducers may be preferred by some for evaluation of shallow organs such as the pancreas, where the depth of tissue penetration is less critical [3]. Similarly, sectoral transducers may be more suited to the precise examination of tubular structures using only a limited area of contact, such as the common bile duct during laparoscopic cholecystectomy (Fig. 5.3), or vascular structures following arterial reconstructions. Inevitably, the need for more than a single transducer will increase the overall cost of the system.

Some manufacturers have also sought to improve access to certain areas of the abdomen by designing flexible laparoscopic ultrasound probes, or probes with movable transducers (Fig. 5.4). However, so far we remain un-

Fig. 5.3 Transverse laparoscopic sonogram through the hepatoduodenal ligament using a 90° sector-scanning probe during laparoscopic cholecystectomy. Near-field imaging is optimal and the tubular structures are precisely localised beneath the probe tip (insert). CBD, common bile duct; HA, heptic artery; PV, portal vein.

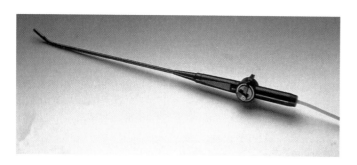

Fig. 5.4 Linear-array laparoscopic ultrasound probe with a flexible transducer tip manipulated from the handpiece. (Courtesy of Tetrad Inc.)

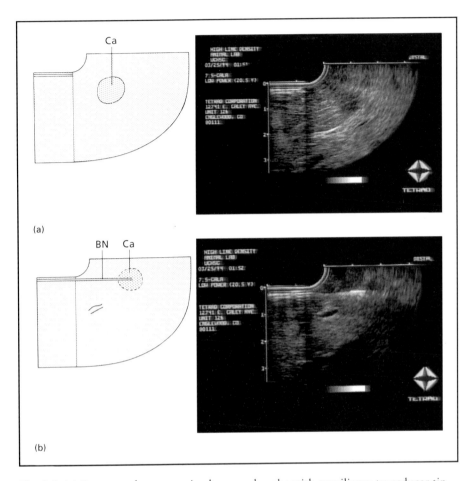

Fig. 5.5 (a) Prototype laparoscopic ultrasound probe with curvilinear transducer tip allowing forward/oblique viewing, and (b) precise placement of biopsy needle (BN) into a hypoechoic carcinoma (Ca). (Courtesy of Tetrad Inc.)

certain of their necessity in the laparoscopic ultrasound assessment of the organs of the upper abdomen. The liver, biliary system and pancreas can invariably be examined thoroughly using a rigid ultrasound probe, and if improved transducer contact with uneven or curved surfaces is desired, this may be achieved by appropriate port positioning, the instillation of fluid into the abdomen or desufflation of the pneumoperitoneum. Flexible probes diminish tactile feedback compared with rigid probes, and the laparoscopic ultrasonographer's attention may be distracted from the examination by the need for continuing manipulation of the articulating probe. The surgeon attempting to acquire experience in laparoscopic ultrasonography and at the bottom end of the learning curve may find the increased complexity of a flexible probe a more daunting proposition than a rigid wand. None the less, it may be that a probe with a movable transducer at the tip will facilitate laparoscopic ultrasound targeted biopsy. The incorporation of a biopsy channel within the shaft of the laparoscopic ultrasound probe, whereby a needle may be reproducibly introduced into the beam of the deflected transducer, may permit accurate and reproducible placement of biopsy needles

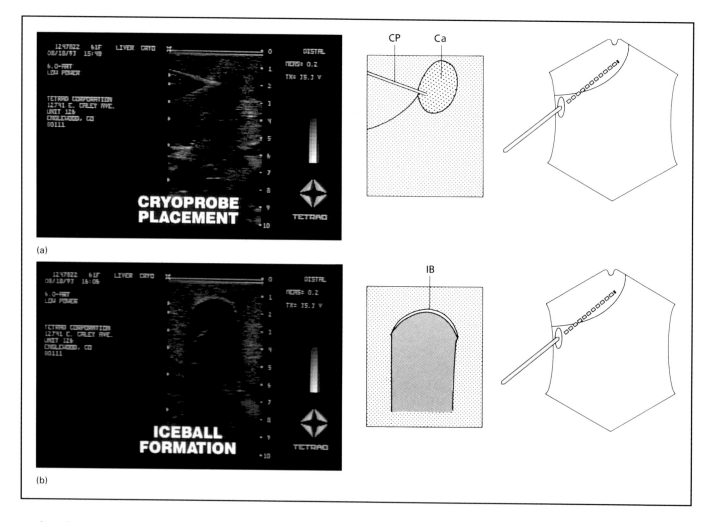

within deep-seated lesions. This type of system might also facilitate the delivery of interstitial therapy to the liver at the same time as the laparoscopic intra-abdominal tumour staging. However, current attempts at producing a laparoscopic ultrasound guided needle biopsy system have utilised a prototype linear-array transducer which features a curvilinear termination to the transducer tip, thus allowing two-dimensional imaging in both forward and sideways directions. The incorporation of a spring-loaded core-cutting biopsy needle within a channel in the rigid probe shaft allows the needle tip to be accurately introduced into the target lesion under direct vision in the forward viewing plane (Figs 5.5 and 5.6).

Further refinements include the provision of a remote control handpiece which may be placed within a sterile bag, thereby transferring control of the ultrasound machine to the operating ultrasonographer.

Developments in ultrasound technology continue to be made and adapted for intraoperative or laparoscopic use. Nevertheless, it is important that a sense of perspective is maintained, and that both the surgeon and the manufacturers do not become obsessed with the imagery of intraoperative and laparoscopic ultrasonography. Existing ultrasound machines and transducers are competitively priced and more than adequate to enable the surgeon

Fig. 5.6 Laparoscopic ultrasound guided cryotherapy of a hypoechoic liver tumour (Ca). (a) The cryoprobe (CP) is directed under guidance into the centre of the lesion, and the freezing of the lesion monitored sonographically. (b) The ice ball (IB) demonstrates a hyperechoic rim and casts a dense posterior acoustic shadow. (Courtesy of Tetrad Inc.)

to make clinically relevant decisions on patients with hepatobiliary and pancreatic disorders. Intraoperative and laparoscopic ultrasonography will remain widely accepted as clinically useful diagnostic modalities on condition that the equipment remains affordable, user-friendly and capable of delivering satisfactory images.

Indications

The explosion of interest in minimal access surgery and the advent of laparoscopic ultrasonography will undoubtedly stimulate more interest in invasive contact ultrasonographic techniques amongst surgeons. Some may even consider adopting transcutaneous ultrasonography as an out-patient or ward-based procedure. It has been shown that such techniques may be rapidly learned by surgeons in training and successfully applied in clinical surgical practice [4].

Intraoperative ultrasonography has been exploited in a number of specialities apart from hepatobiliary and pancreatic surgery, and the indications for its use remain very diverse.

Endocrine surgery

Endocrine surgeons have employed this technology during operations for neuroendocrine neoplasia in and around the pancreas. Galiber *et al.* [5] demonstrated the superior sensitivity of operative palpation and intraoperative sonography in the detection of insulinomas compared with preoperative ultrasonography, computerised tomography (CT) scanning and angiography (see also Chapter 4). Kern *et al.* [6] have also reported the advantages of intraoperative ultrasound during operations for parathyroid disease. They demonstrated that intraoperative ultrasonography using a 7.5–10-MHz curvilinear-array probe was both more sensitive and demonstrated a superior positive predictive value compared with preoperative imaging investigations (CT scanning, scintigraphy, transcutaneous ultrasonography) in localising abnormal parathyroid glands during reoperative neck surgery [6].

Vascular surgery

Before the advent of contemporary B-mode imaging probes, intraoperative ultrasound during vascular reconstructive surgery relied upon velocity signal analysis and the subjective appreciation of audible Doppler signals obtained with the Doppler probe held in proximity to the reconstructed vascular segment [7]. This principle has since been extended to the use of high-resolution intraoperative duplex Doppler ultrasonography as a 'quality control' measure in the detection of technical defects following carotid endarterectomy [8], renal artery revascularisation procedures [9] and in a variety of peripheral arterial bypass procedures [10,11]. Similarly, the patency and quality of vascular anastomoses may be readily assessed during organ

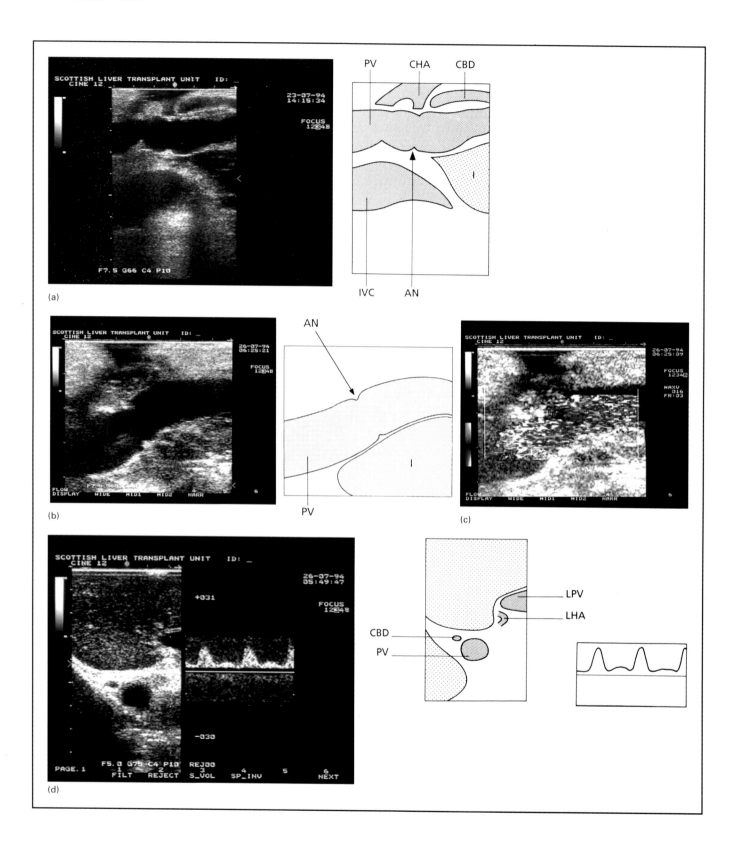

(a)

(b)

(c)

(d)

transplantation procedures, giving the opportunity for early corrective intervention with the recognition of anastamotic defects or inadequate graft inflow [12] (Fig. 5.7). Intraoperative duplex ultrasound techniques employing Doppler spectral analysis and quantitative flow measurements generally require the presence of a properly trained assistant or vascular technician in the operating theatre. A detailed description of these techniques are beyond the scope of this book and readers are referred to more specialist texts [9,13–15].

Urology

As might be expected from the experiences of biliary surgeons who recognised the utility of contact ultrasonography in the detection of choledocholithiasis during cholecystectomy, this technique has also been found to be useful in the detection and localisation of renal calculi during nephrolithotomy [16]. The benefits of this approach also include the ability to define avascular areas suitable for incision without the need for renal artery clamping. Although this approach to the management of nephrolithiasis has waned in favour of alternative non-invasive and minimal access techniques, it is feasible that intraoperative and laparoscopic ultrasonography may prove useful in the management of patients with large staghorn calculi who require operative intervention.

Neurosurgery

The value of intraoperative ultrasonography in both intracranial neurosurgical procedures and during spinal surgery has been well documented [17,18]. It is possible to image all types of brain tumour well, and abscesses, vascular malformations and structural defects may be defined. Intraoperative sonography is ideal for the precise localisation of both deep-seated and superficial lesions, and the guidance of their biopsy or aspiration.

Fig. 5.7 (*Facing page*) Intraoperative sonogram using a 7.5-MHz linear-array T-probe performed following the completion of an orthotopic liver transplant. (a,b) The reconstructed infrahepatic vena cava (IVC), portal vein (PV), common bile duct (CBD) and common hepatic artery (CHA) are depicted in their long axes with the caudate lobe of the allograft demonstrated posteriorly (I). The PV anastamosis (AN) is seen as a slightly elevated hyperechoic ridge on the luminal aspect of the vessel (arrowed). (c) Colour Doppler flow enhancement immediately demonstrates laminar high flow in the PV with no obstruction or turbulence. (d) Transverse sonogram through the porta hepatis demonstrating the left portal vein (LPV) and artery (LPA). Doppler sampling of the left hepatic artery (LHA) has demonstrated a good arterial signal confirming satisfactory flow upstream of the hepatic artery anastamosis. The probe position used in (a–c) is the same as that used in Fig. 2.9. The probe position used in (d) is the same as that used in Fig. 3.32(a,b).

Surgical gastroenterology

A number of surgeons have already established the potential of intraoperative ultrasonography as a means of improving the staging of gastrointestinal malignancies at open operation, and several authors have testified to the sensitivity of routine intraoperative ultrasonography in the detection of 'occult' hepatic metastases in patients undergoing apparently curative resection of both colorectal carcinomas [19–25], and a variety of other primary gastrointestinal tumours [26]. It is now apparent that tumour staging can be considerably improved by the addition of ultrasonography to staging laparoscopy in a variety of circumstances. Our own experience has highlighted both its application and its influence on clinical decision making in patients with pancreatic and hepatobiliary malignancy.

In other fields of clinical practice the advantages may not yet be so obvious. The rationale for laparoscopic staging of oesophagogastric malignancy is well established [27–30], and the addition of laparoscopic ultrasonography may improve the detection of hepatic metastases. Machi *et al.* [31,32] have reported their ability, using high-resolution intraoperative ultrasonography, to define the five discrete echo-layers of the stomach wall, and so accurately determine the T-stage and precise depth of mural tumour invasion in patients with oesophagogastric carcinoma. They found that operative ultrasound was able to detect tumours that were otherwise impalpable, and that similarly, lateral tumour extension in the stomach wall was more accurately defined than by palpation. Extramural local tumour invasion of oesophageal cancer, especially to the adjacent blood vessels, was more accurately assessed than by preoperative imaging methods [31]. Our preliminary experience has indicated that this information is also readily obtained with staging laparoscopic ultrasonography (Fig. 5.8). The examination may also be used to demonstrate regional lymph node involvement by tumour. Although this information may not prevent the surgeon contemplating a palliative resection of the tumour to deal with obstructive or haemorrhagic symptoms, full preoperative staging in this way undoubtedly renders him/her better equipped to make rational decisions on the need for adjuvant therapy at an earlier stage, and concerning the planned extent of resectional surgery.

For those contemplating hepatic resection by laparoscopic means [33], it would seem logical that the vascular anatomy be identified by laparoscopic ultrasound before any dissection is undertaken.

It is not yet clear whether laparoscopic assisted resection of colorectal malignancy is likely to become established in clinical practice. If this proves to be the case, laparoscopic ultrasonography will prove to be indispensable in performing a full intra-abdominal staging of the disease, given the surgeon's loss of tactile feedback and inability to palpate adequately the liver. As indicated earlier, many authors have demonstrated the sensitivity of intraoperative ultrasound over and above manual palpation in the detection of occult liver metastases at open operation. Although the use of color Dop-

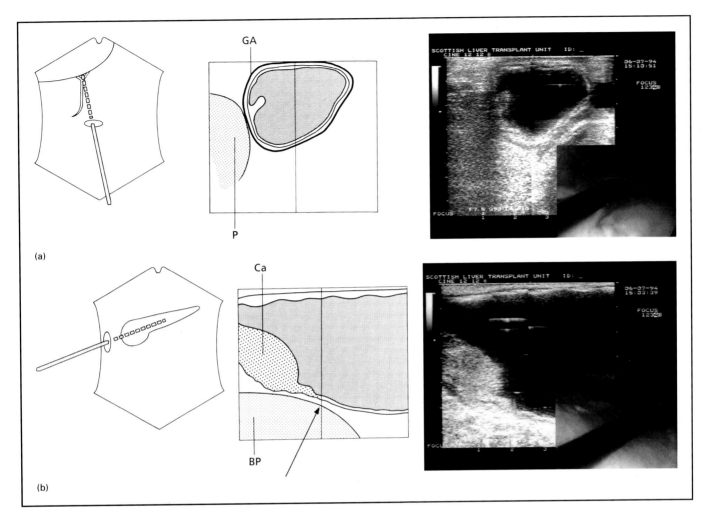

Fig. 5.8 (a) A sagittal laparoscopic sonogram through the gastric antrum (GA) demonstrates the individual echo-layers of the stomach wall which appear normal at this level. (b) When the probe (P) is positioned obliquely in the long axis of the stomach an exophytic gastric carcinoma (Ca) is demonstrated protruding into the lumen of the gastric fundus. The superior extent of the Ca is demonstrated where the stomach wall retains its normal structure superiorly (arrowed). The examination is facilitated by the instillation of 1 L of saline into the stomach via the nasogastric tube which appears as a hyperechoic artefact within the gastric lumen. BP, body of the pancreas.

pler intraoperative ultrasound in the localisation of the ureter has been described [34], it seems unlikely that laparoscopic ultrasonography will find popularity as an aid to defining the anatomy during colorectal surgery.

Some workers have attempted to further improve the sensitivity of high-resolution intraoperative ultrasound in the detection of both primary and secondary liver tumours by the administration of echo-contrast agents into the hepatic circulation. Takada *et al.* [35] injected carbon dioxide gas into the hepatic artery of patients under investigation for impalpable hepatocellular carcinoma. They were able to demonstrate small tumours in two out of nine patients which were otherwise undetectable by non-enhanced ultrasonography. Conversely, El Mouaaouy *et al.* [36] injected the agent SHU 454 via the portal vein or common bile duct in to patients with both primary and secondary liver lesions, describing improvement in their ability to detect the tumours in certain cases. More recently, Leen *et al.* [37] described the apparent advantage of administering galactose microparticles intravenously in order to improve the sensitivity of transcutaneous colour Doppler ultrasonography in the detection of colorectal liver metastases. However, it remains to be seen whether this approach will become a worthwhile adjunct to high-resolution contact ultrasonography in the evaluation of the liver.

Pelvic surgery

In the field of gynaecology, some workers have already recognised the potential for laparoscopic ultrasound assessment of the adequacy of endometrial curettage (Fig. 5.9). It may be that urologists and others will wish to apply this technology in similar ways.

Thoracic surgery

Staging cervical mediastinoscopy with mediastinal ultrasonography has recently been advocated in the preoperative management of patients with lung cancer [38]. Mediastinal ultrasonography was shown to be superior to thoracic CT scanning in the diagnosis of malignant mediastinal lymphadenopathy by measuring the short-axis dimension of the nodes. Subcarinal lymph nodes which were inaccessible to cervical mediastinoscopy could be identified and safe biopsy achieved [38].

Professional issues

There will remain considerable debate as to which clinician is best qualified to undertake operative and laparoscopic ultrasonography. Whereas the radiologist may have detailed knowledge of abdominal ultrasonography, it seems likely that the individual undertaking the operative procedure will be best able to undertake the ultrasound evaluation. It may be that the surgeon will require the assistance of an ultrasound expert in the early stages, but our own experience suggests that the learning curve is not particularly long and that from a practical point of view the surgeon is unlikely to have available the regular support of a radiologist. Similarly, we have on several occa-

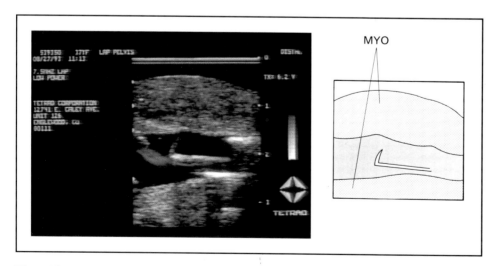

Fig. 5.9 Laparoscopic sonogram demonstrating endometrial curettage with the surgical scraper inserted within the uterine lumen, hook facing upwards. MYO, myometrium. (Courtesy of Tetrad Inc.)

sions found that the anatomical definition is such that the surgeon, with his/her detailed knowledge of the anatomy, is better equipped to interpret the images.

It should be borne in mind that the actual procedure of intraoperative or laparoscopic ultrasonography does not expose the patient to any additional risk and that the information obtained from the laparoscopic examination alone may be invaluable. As for many laparoscopic procedures, the technique is probably best learnt by proctoring. We have used 1- and 2-day courses to introduce the technique to surgeons. Unlike most laparoscopic surgery it is a difficult technique to learn on simulators and the skills are best acquired first-hand during open and laparoscopic procedures. In our experience, laparoscopic cholecystectomy has proved an ideal opportunity for the surgeon to spend a limited amount of time to learn the technique. In this way there is no pressure on the surgeon that a failure to detect an abnormality will influence the operative decision making. It may be appropriate to defer assessment of cancer patients until such time as the surgeon is confident in interpreting the images. However, as has been demonstrated from our own experience the information obtained from diagnostic laparoscopy should give the surgeon confidence to extend the examination to include an ultrasound examination.

References

1 Grant EG, Schiller VL, Millener P, *et al*. Color Doppler imaging of the hepatic vasculature. *Am J Roentgenol* 1992; 159: 943–50.

2 Yamashita Y, Kurohiji T, Hayashi J, Kimitsuki H, Hiraki M, Kakegawa T. Intraoperative ultrasonography during laparoscopic cholecystectomy. *Surg Laparosc Endosc* 1993; 3: 167–71.

3 John TG, Garden OJ. Clinical experience with sector scan and linear array ultrasound probes in laparoscopic surgery. *Endosc Surg Allied Technol* 1994; 2: 134–42.

4 Williams RJL, Mann DV, Windsor ACJ, Crofton M, Rosin RD. Ultrasound scanning of the acute abdomen by surgeons in training. *Ann Roy Col Surg Engl* 1994; 76: 228–33.

5 Galiber AK, Reading CC, Charboneau JW, *et al*. Localisation of pancreatic insulinoma: comparison of pre- and intraoperative US with CT and angiography. *Radiology* 1988; 166: 405–8.

6 Kern KA, Shawker TH, Doppman JL, *et al*. The use of high resolution ultrasound to locate parathyroid tumors during reoperations for primary hyperparathyroidism. *World J Surg* 1987; 11: 579–85.

7 Barnes R, Garrett WV. Intraoperative assessment of arterial reconstruction by Doppler ultrasound. *Sorg Gyn Obst* 1978; 146: 896–900.

8 Hoff C, de Gier P, Buth J. Intraoperative duplex monitoring of the carotid bifurcation for the detection of technical defects. *Eur J Vasc Surg* 1994; 8: 441–7.

9 Lantz EJ, Charboneau JW, Hallet JW, Dougherty MJ, James EM. Intraoperative color Doppler sonography during renal artery revascularisation. *Am J Roentgenol* 1994; 162: 859–63.

10 Sigel B, Coelho JCU, Flanigan DP, Schuler JJ, Machi J, Beitler JC. Detection of vascular defects during operation by imaging ultrasound. *Ann Surg* 1982; 196: 473–80.

11 Rosenbloom MS, Flanigan DP. The use of ultrasound during reconstructive arterial surgery of the lower extremities. *World J Surg* 1987; 11: 598–603.

12 Bismuth H, Kuntslinger F, Castaing D. Ultrasound and liver transplantation. In: Bismuth H, Kuntslinger F, Castaing D, eds. *A Text and Atlas of Liver Ultrasound.* London: Chapman and Hall, 1991: 126–35.

13 Sigel B, Machi J, Flanigan DP, Schuler JJ. Intraoperative B-mode ultrasound techniques for arterial evaluation. In: Zweibel WJ, ed. *Introduction to Vascular Ultrasonography,* 2nd edn. New York: Grune and Stratton, 1986: 474–84.

14 Lane RJ, Ackroyd N, Appleberg M, Graham J. The application of operative ultrasound following carotid endarterectomy. *World J Surg* 1987; 11: 593–7.

15 Lefor AT, Flowers JL. Laparoscopic wedge biopsy of the liver. *J Am Col Surg* 1994; 178: 307–8.

16 Alken P, Thüroff JW, Hammer C. The use of operative ultrasonography for the localisation of renal calculi. *World J Surg* 1987; 11: 586–92.

17 Chandler WF, Rubin JM. The application of ultrasound during brain surgery. *World J Surg* 1987; 11: 558–69.

18 Rubin JM, Chandler WF. The use of ultrasound during spinal cord surgery. *World J Surg* 1987; 11: 570–8.

19 Charnley RM, Morris DL, Dennison AR, Amar SS, Hardcastle JD. Improved detection of colorectal liver metastases by intra-operative ultrasound. *Br J Surg* 1988; 75: 1262 (Abstract).

20 Stadler J, Hölscher AH, Adolf J. Intraoperative ultrasonographic detection of occult liver metastases in colorectal cancer. *Surg Endosc* 1991; 5: 36–40.

21 Machi J, Isomoto H, Kurohiji T, *et al.* Accuracy of intraoperative ultrasound in diagnosing liver metastasis from colorectal cancer: evaluation with postoperative follow-up results. *World J Surg* 1991; 15: 551–7.

22 Boldrini G, de Gaetano AM, Giovannini I, Castagneto M, Colagrande C, Castiglioni G. The systematic use of operative ultrasound for detection of liver metastases during colorectal surgery. *World J Surg* 1987; 11: 622–7.

23 Gozzetti G, Mazziotti A, Bolondi L, *et al.* Intraoperative ultrasonography in surgery for liver tumours. *Surgery* 1986; 99: 523–9.

24 Stone MD, Kane R, Bothe A, Jessup JM, Cady B, Steele GD. Intraoperative ultrasound imaging of the liver at the time of colorectal cancer resection. *Arch Surg* 1994; 129: 431–6.

25 Olsen AK. Intraoperative ultrasonography and the detection of liver metastases in patients with colorectal cancer. *Br J Surg* 1990; 77: 998–9.

26 Machi J, Sigel B, Zaren HA, Kurohiji T, Yamashita Y. Operative ultrasonography during hepatobiliary and pancreatic surgery. *World J Surg* 1993; 17: 640–6.

27 Shandall A, Johnson C. Laparoscopy or scanning in oesophageal and gastric carcinoma. *Br J Surg* 1985; 72: 449–51.

28 Possik RA, Franco EL, Pires DR, Wohnrath DR, Ferreira EB. Sensitivity, specificity, and predictive value of laparoscopy for the staging of gastric cancer and for the detection of liver metastases. *Cancer* 1986; 58: 1–6.

29 Gross E, Bancewicz J, Ingram G. Assessment of gastric carcinoma by laparoscopy. *Br Med J* 1984; 288: 1577.

30 Watt I, Stewart I, Anderson D, Bell G, Anderson JR. Laparoscopy, ultrasound and computed tomography in cancer of the oesophagus and gastric cardia: a prospective comparison for detecting intra-abdominal metastases. *Br J Surg* 1989; 76: 1036–9.

31 Machi J, Takeda J, Sigel B, Kakegawa T. Normal stomach wall and gastric cancer: evaluation with high-resolution operative US. *Radiology* 1986; 159: 85–8.

32 Machi J, Takeda J, Kakegawa T, *et al.* The detection of gastric and esophageal tumor extension by high-resolution ultrasound during surgery. *World J Surg* 1987; 11: 664–71.

33 Katkhouda N, Mouiel J. Laparoscopic surgery of the liver. In: Cuesta MA, Nagy AG, eds. *Minimally Invasive Surgery in Gastrointestinal Cancer.* Edinburgh: Churchill Livingstone, 1993: 81–93.

34 Smith LE, Wherry D, Marohn M. Use of ultrasound to identify the ureter. *Surg Endosc* 1993; 8: 467.

35 Takada T, Yasuda H, Uchiyama K, Hasegawa H, Shikata J. Contrast-enhanced intraoperative ultrasonography of small hepatocellular carcinomas. *Surgery* 1990; 107: 528–32.

36 El Mouaaouy A, Naruhn M, Becker HD, Schlief R. Intraoperative echo-contrast ultrasound examination of malignant liver neoplasms—initial clinical experience. *Surg Endosc* 1991; 5: 214–18.

37 Leen E, Angerson WJ, Warren HW, *et al.* Improved sensitivity of colour Doppler flow imaging of colorectal hepatic metastases using galactose microparticles: a preliminary report. *Br J Surg* 1994; 81: 252–4.

38 Nakano N, Nakahara K, Yasumitsu T, Kotake Y, Ikezoe J, Kawashima Y. Mediastinal ultrasonography for the assessment of mediastinal lymph node metastases in lung cancer patients. *Surg Today (Jpn J Surg)* 1994; 24: 106–11.

Index